AF327793

Treatable and Potentially Preventable Dementias

Treatable and Potentially Preventable Dementias

Edited by

Vladimir Hachinski
University of Western Ontario

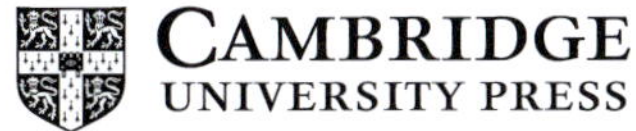

CAMBRIDGE
UNIVERSITY PRESS

University Printing House, Cambridge CB2 8BS, United Kingdom

One Liberty Plaza, 20th Floor, New York, NY 10006, USA

477 Williamstown Road, Port Melbourne, VIC 3207, Australia

314–321, 3rd Floor, Plot 3, Splendor Forum, Jasola District Centre, New Delhi – 110025, India

79 Anson Road, #06–04/06, Singapore 079906

Cambridge University Press is part of the University of Cambridge.

It furthers the University's mission by disseminating knowledge in the pursuit of education, learning, and research at the highest international levels of excellence.

www.cambridge.org
Information on this title: www.cambridge.org/9781107157460
DOI: 10.1017/9781316662007

First published 2018

Printed in the United Kingdom by TJ International Ltd. Padstow Cornwall

A catalogue record for this publication is available from the British Library.

Library of Congress Cataloging-in-Publication Data
Names: Hachinski, Vladimir, editor.
Title: Treatable and potentially preventable dementias / edited by Vladimir Hachinski.
Description: New York : Cambridge University Press, 2018. | Includes bibliographical references and index.
Identifiers: LCCN 2017055357| ISBN 9781107157460 (hardback : alk. paper) | ISBN 9781316662007 (Cambridge Core)
Subjects: | MESH: Dementia – diagnosis | Dementia – prevention & control | Cognitive Dysfunction | Stroke – complications
Classification: LCC RC521 | NLM WM 220 | DDC 616.8/31–dc23
LC record available at https://lccn.loc.gov/2017055357

ISBN 978-1-107-15746-0 Hardback

....

Contents

Contributors

Mahmoud Reza Azarpazhooh, MD
Department of Neurology, Ghaem
Hospital,
Mashhad University of Medical Sciences,
Mashhad, Iran

Michael Brainin, MD, FESO, FAHA
Professor in Clinical Neurology,
Department for Clinical Neurosciences and
Preventive Medicine, Danube University,
Krems, Austria

Vladimir Hachinski, MD, DSc, FAHA
Distinguished University Professor
Department of Clinical Neurological
Sciences,
London Health Sciences Centre,
University of Western Ontario, Ontario,
Canada

Krister Håkansson, PhD
Department of Neurobiology, Care
Sciences and Society, Division of
Clinical Geriatrics, Karolinska Institute,
Stockholm, Sweden
Department of Psychology,
Linnaeus University, Kalmar,
Sweden

Lawrence S. Honig, MD, PhD
Professor of Neurology at Columbia
University Medical Center,
Taub Institute for Research on Alzheimer's
Disease and the Aging Brain,
Gertrude H. Sergievsky Center (PH19) and
Department of Neurology
Columbia University College of Physicians
& Surgeons
New York, USA

Miia Kivipelto, MD, PhD
Department of Neurobiology, Care
Sciences and Society, Division of Clinical

Geriatrics, Karolinska Institute, Stockholm,
Sweden
Department of Neurology, University of
Eastern Finland, Kuopio,
Finland

Antonia Nucera, MD
Neurology Stroke Unit
Fabrizio Spaziani Hospital, Frosinone,
Italy

José G. Merino, MD, MPhil
Associate Professor, Department of
Neurology,
University of Maryland School of Medicine,
Baltimore, MD, USA

Tiia Ngandu, PhD
Department of Chronic Disease
Prevention,
National Institute for Health and Welfare
Helsinki, Finland

J. David Spence, MD, FRPC, FAHA
Stroke Prevention & Atherosclerosis
Research Centre,
Robarts Research Institute, Western
University,
Ontario, Canada

Yvonne Teuschl, PhD
Assistant Professor, Department for
Clinical Neurosciences and Preventive
Medicine, Danube University, Krems,
Austria

Clinton B. Wright, MD, MS
Associate Director, NINDS
Director, Division of Clinical Research
National Institute of Neurological
Disorders and Stroke
Neuroscience Center
Bethesda, MD USA

Foreword

An accompaniment of increases in life expectancy is demographic aging and growth in the number of persons with dementia. Worldwide, it is estimated that there are 47 million persons with dementia, and by the year 2050 it is expected that this number will reach over 130 million. Dementia exacts a high financial and personal toll. In the United States, the yearly per person monetary cost attributable to dementia is in the range of US $41,000 to $56,000 with a total estimated annual cost of up to $215 billion. The expected rise in the number of persons in the community with cognitive impairment and dementia places substantial challenges on the delivery of medical and other services, and on family members who are tasked with caregiving responsibilities. As the "super-aging" phenomenon continues in developed countries, innovative public health policy will be needed to address housing, user-friendly community environments, and specially tailored community services to help improve the quality of life of our elderly and those with cognitive impairment and dementia.

Over time, a major shift in scientific thought is being embraced by some in relation to how we conceptualize dementias of later life, such as Alzheimer disease and vascular cognitive impairment, and a number of the leading causes of mortality. Thanks in large part to the insight and work of Vladimir Hachinski, we acknowledge shared common mechanistic pathways of inflammation and oxidative stress that link many of the leading causes of mortality including the dementias, the importance of lifestyle and traditional cardiovascular risks for many of these same diseases, the common finding of a vascular component in the major dementias, and the importance of screening for vascular risks and treating them. Thus, major dementias may be preventable.

Treatable and Potentially Preventable Dementias provides a refreshing viewpoint and paves the way for a major shift in how we think about dementias of later life and manage them. One will need to discard nosologic "bucket thinking" (i.e., neurodegenerative versus vascular classification buckets) and join those who have moved mechanistically upstream to the "brain-at-risk" stage to intervene. An excellent example of potential preventability of cognitive impairment is the Finnish Geriatric Intervention Study to Prevent Cognitive Impairment and Disability (FINGER). This multidomain intervention, designed to maintain cognitive vitality, included at-risk elderly in the general population and resulted in hope to slow or prevent cognitive decline by vascular risk modification. *Treatable and Potentially Preventable Dementias* will challenge practitioners to approach dementias of later life in a different manner. The text comes on the heels of an Institute of Medicine (IOM) report on understanding progress and opportunities for action in cognitive aging to preserve brain health. The IOM report emphasizes physical activity and management of cardiovascular risks to help maintain cognitive vitality.

Treatable and Potentially Preventable Dementias, edited by Vladimir Hachinski, a visionary, is written by many well-known scientists in the field, and is timely and authoritative. It is a foremost textbook in the field as it explores means to maintain brain health. The book provides a practical format for transfer of information and is designed for those who deal with stroke, cognitive impairment, or both.

Philip B. Gorelick

Preface

Cerebrovascular disease and Alzheimer disease often occur together, but are studied apart. Stroke physicians have yet to embrace the fact that most cerebrovascular disease is asymptomatic, affecting not the body but the mind. Similarly, dementia doctors have yet to acknowledge that all major dementias have a vascular component, ranging from 61 percent in frontotemporal dementia to 80 percent in Alzheimer disease, which doubles the chances of silent brain pathology manifesting as dementia. This creates a wide gap between what we know and what is applied, offering a great opportunity to make a difference. This book aims to help fill the gap and realize the opportunity.

We also address the neglected topic of treatable components of dementia, enlarging the range of what physicians can do for their patients. Our approach is founded on a simple premise: of all the common mechanisms of dementia, the only treatable and preventable one is the vascular. The vascular cognitive impairment approach consists of identifying the vascular risk and protective factors, beginning with the asymptomatic "brain at risk" stage, through to the warning, and stroke stage and in individuals with cognitive impairment.

The book is aimed at neurologists, geriatricians, internists, psychiatrists, physiatrists, general practitioners, and all physicians dealing with stroke, dementia, and those at risk for both. We begin with a review of the basics, describe typical patients and presentations, and provide clear guidelines in diagnoses, management, and prevention. Extensive figures, tables, and diagrams complement the text and ease understanding. Although the book rests on an extensive scientific background, the main facts and conclusions are presented in a summarized, practical manner meant to be applied for the benefit of a growing number of patients.

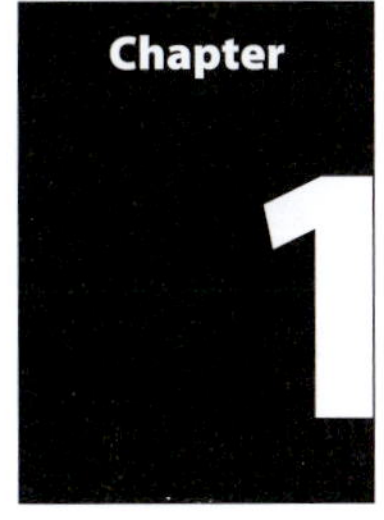

Chapter 1

Pathophysiology & Epidemiology

Mahmoud Reza Azarpazhooh and Vladimir Hachinski

Perspective

Once upon a time things were simple. Increasing age hardened the brain arteries, causing a slow strangulation of the brain's blood supply, resulting in chronic ischemia and neuronal death. However, in the 1970s a number of studies demonstrated that when vascular disease was responsible for dementia, it most often acted through the agency of cerebral infarcts, which led to the concept of "multi infarct dementia" meaning that it resulted from multiple cerebral infarcts large and small.[1] This stricter definition of vascular dementia contributed to the impression that cerebrovascular disease was an uncommon cause of dementia.

Hitherto, Alzheimer disease had been considered a pre-senile dementia and rare. However, with the waning of "atherosclerotic dementia" as the main cause of cognitive decline and increasing concern about cognitive impairment in the elderly, an expert committee developed criteria for "Alzheimer disease" in the elderly.[2] Although at the time, it was not clear whether the hallmark lesions of pre-senile dementia, namely plaques and neurofibrillary tangles, that also appear in the elderly represented the same process, a controversy that remains to this day.

This chapter provides a brief overview of basic anatomy and physiology of the brain, a description of cognitive abilities and their relevant age-related changes, and finally, the importance of vascular cognitive impairment.

Basic Anatomy and Physiology

Undoubtedly, the brain is by far the most complex organ. It contains 10^{11} neurons and at least 1000 dendrites per neuron, producing an extremely extensive network of billions of nerve cells, enabling human beings to perform a wide range of activities, from autonomic responses to higher cognitive functions of memory and thought.[3] Not surprisingly, the brain is also one of the most metabolically demanding organs in the human body. Due to the lack of long-term substrate storage and a very high rate of metabolic demand, it needs a continuous supply of blood and oxygen.[4,5] Moreover, the optimal function of the brain cells is only possible in a stable microenvironment, independent of the changes in the periphery. Such strict homeostatic control is achieved via a blood-brain barrier (BBB) and in a special unit of neurons, glia, and vascular tissues: the "neurovascular unit."

The Difference between White Matter and Grey Matter

The brain is divided into grey (substantia grisea) and white matter (substantia alba). It is an extremely interconnected organ, where each and every neuron within the grey matter connects between 1000 to 10000 nearby neurons, and at the same time, long-distance

1

communication between neurons at separate brain locations is mediated via the white matter.[6]

The grey matter consists of nerve cell bodies, their dendrites and local ramifications of axons, glial cells, and blood vessels. On the other hand, the white matter is made up of bundles of myelinated axons, trafficking in and out of the grey matter and connecting mostly separated cortical regions rather than the cortical to adjacent subcortical structures.[7,8] Long-range myelinated axon tracts with relatively few cell bodies in the white matter and numerous cell bodies with relatively few myelinated axons in the grey matter lead to distinctive color of white and grey in the brain.

Not surprisingly, larger brains, such as human's brains, require longer fibers to communicate, and consequently the volume of the white matter that increases disproportionately faster than the volume of the grey matter.[7] However, the brain's white matter, with almost 50 percent of total brain volume, consumes less energy than grey matter. This is partially due to the dramatically lower number of synapses (if any) in white matter, since the highest level of energy in the brain is used to provide appropriate neuronal connections via synapses.

Although traditionally a majority of cognitive functions are attributed to grey matter, it was clearly shown that age-related cognitive decline in healthy older individuals may happen due to characteristic changes in the ultrastructure of myelin coupled with evidence of inflammatory processes in the white matter.[9] The white matter is quite vulnerable to a broad range of neurological diseases, such as cerebral ischemia and dementing processes. The myelin in the white matter is formed by oligodendrocytes, one of the most vulnerable cells in the brain. Moreover, blood flow and cerebrovascular reactivity in the cerebral cortex of young subjects are significantly higher than those for the white matter in the elderly.[10] It varies based on the type of brain tissues and age, ranging from 20ml/100g/min in white matter to 70/100g/min in grey matter, and is higher in neonates and infants than in adults.[4,11] Impaired autoregulation and higher levels of cerebrovascular resistance were also significantly more prevalent in patients with periventricular white matter lesions,[12] increasing substantially the risk of dementia in elderly people.[13]

The Neurovascular Unit

The BBB is a highly selective permeability barrier, separating the central nervous system (CNS) from the peripheral circulation and plays a critical role in the maintenance of CNS homeostasis. This regulatory interface includes three major components, namely the BBB-endothelial cells, astrocyte end-feet, and pericytes (Figure 1.1).[14,15] Tight junctions between endothelial cells (about 50–100 times tighter than peripheral microvessels), the absence of intercellular clefts, lack of fenestrations, minor pinocytic activity, and a high transendothelial electrical resistance contribute significantly in the selective function of BBB and provide a strict homeostatic control over the brain.[16,17] From one side, the BBB is supported by astrocytes and pericytes, and from the other side it is closely connected to microglia and neurons.[18,19] This combination of cerebral microvascular endothelium with astrocytes, pericytes, neurons, and the extracellular matrix constitutes a special "neurovascular unit" that is essential for the health and function of the CNS.[15] Such controlling gates and special units can act as the best safeguard mechanism, efficiently protecting the brain from any harmful substance, and at the same time, can sufficiently maintain the ionic concentrations of the central nervous system within a narrow range. However, it is also a major obstacle to

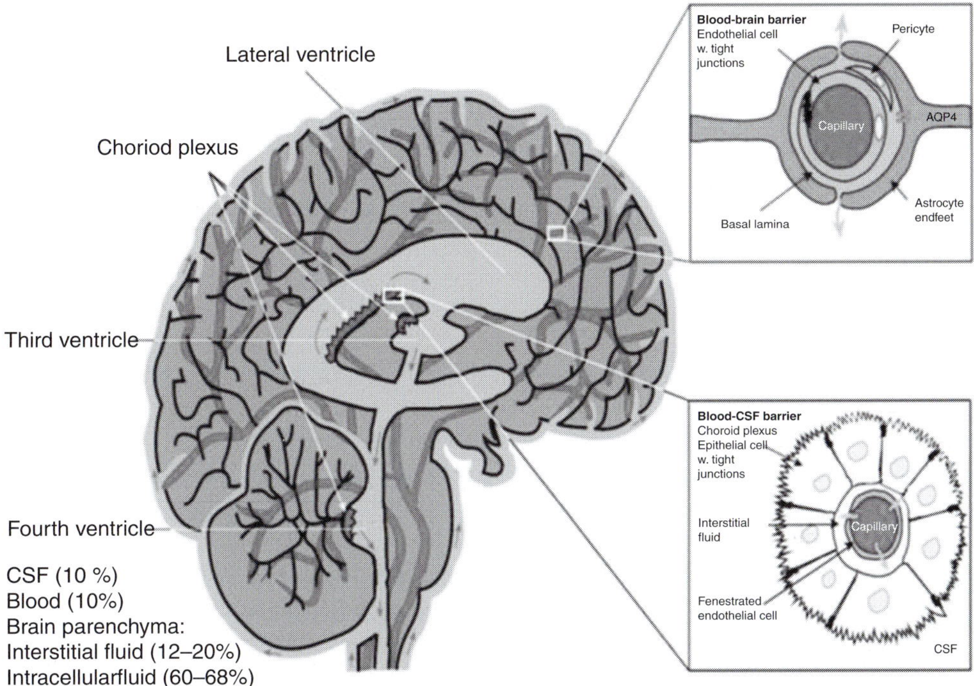

Figure 1.1 Schematic representation of the brain's fluid compartments and barriers. Reproduced by permission of Springer from: Jessen NA, Munk ASF, Lundgaar, I, Nedergaard M. The glymphatic system: a beginner's guide. *Neurochemical Research*. 2015;40(12):1–17.

the delivery of medications to the CNS. Therefore, this barrier can be a friend and simultaneously a foe to clinicians and researchers.[20]

Although the brain has been considered unique due to the lack of a conventional lymphatic system, recently a macroscopic waste clearance system in the brain has been described.[21,22] This is a unique paravascular pathway formed by astroglial cells named the "glymphatic system." This pathway facilitates cerebrospinal flow through the brain parenchyma and the clearance of interstitial solutes and potentially neurotoxic waste products, such as beta amyloid,[21,22] the main component of the amyloid plaques and significant contributors to the pathogenesis of Alzheimer disease.

Cerebral Blood Flow (CBF)

The brain tissues and cells are exquisitely sensitive to oxygen deprivation. Consequently, to meet its optimal requirement, although it only represents 2 percent of body weight, the brain receives almost 15 percent of the body's total cardiac output, approximately 50 ml blood/100g brain tissue /min or 700 ml/min. The blood supply of the brain varies based on the type of brain tissues, ranging from 20ml/100g/min in white matter to 70ml/100g/min in grey matter.[4,11] More important, normal brain function and tissues integrity are highly dependent on the "regulation" for constant supply of oxygen and energy to the brain.[23] Brain blood flow regulation is a process in which, despite the change in cerebral perfusion

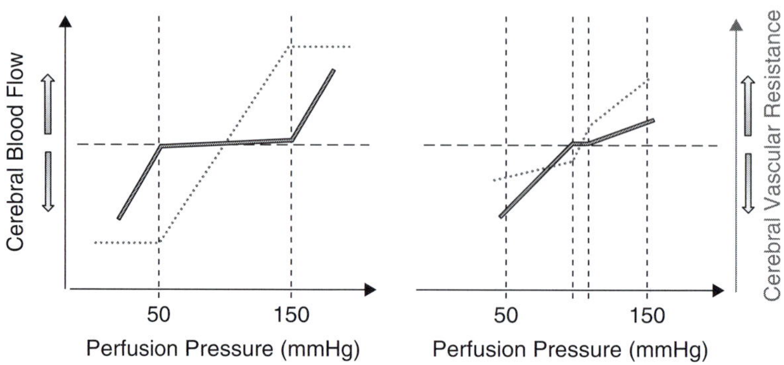

Figure 1.2 The relationship between cerebral blood flow and perfusion pressure. Willie CK., Tzeng Y-C, Fisher J. A, Ainslie PN. Integrative regulation of human brain blood flow. The Journal of Physiology. 2014;592(Pt5):841–859.

pressure (CPP), brain arteries and particularly arterioles, provide a roughly constant amount of CBF to protect the human brain and provide a favorable regional and global oxygen supply to the brain. While autoregulation is also present in other organs of the body, the most developed system is in the brain, where it's regularity maintains a relatively constant amount of blood flow. As shown in Figure 1.2 (left panel), a stable amount of CBF is especially obvious when the mean arterial pressure (MAP) is between ~50 and 150 mm Hg. MAP is a steady component of blood flow during a single cardiac cycle and therefore a better indicator for adequate tissue perfusion, such as the brain than systolic or diastolic pressure. It is calculated as:

$$\text{diastolic pressure} + 1/3 \,(\text{systolic pressure} - \text{diastolic pressure})$$

CBF in MAP above and below these levels becomes completely dependent on MAP in a linear fashion. However, a recent study showed that the CBF–MAP relationship may not be linear through a broad range of MAP (Figure 1.2, right panel).[24]

Knowledge about the patterns and age-associated changes in CBF is an important, yet largely unknown step in the differentiation between the normal aging process and cognitive impairments due to vascular or neurodegenerative diseases.[25] While some studies found that total CBF remains unchanged or decreases minimally during normal aging,[26,27] most researchers find a gradual decline, although at different rates, ranging from 3.9 mL/min[28] to 4.8 mL/min (0.52 percent) per year,[29] and in different anatomical localizations, i.e., grey (0.45 percent to 0.74 percent per year) versus white matter (0.3 percent per year), with increasing age.[30,31]

Cognitive Changes with Aging

Our daily lives depend on the close, coordinated and simultaneous interactions between several cognitive abilities. We need to have adequate attention, be able to collect, memorize, and retrieve relevant information, inhibit distracting or irrelevant information in working memory, make correct decisions, design flexible plans, solve problems appropriately, and perform goal-directed activities. These huge series of mental activities, covering almost all aspects of cognitive functions, logically need to be controlled centrally and coordinated adequately to accomplish any specific task, particularly novel ones, and achieve the desired

Table 1.1 Cognitive domain: classifications, definitions and age-associated changes

	Decline	Remain Stable	Improve
Cognitive functions	Attention Processing speed Short-term memory* Working Memory** (in high demanding tasks) Declarative memory: Episodic memory*** Prospective memory**** Executive function	Decision-making Non-declarative memory: Procedural motor skills[†] Non-declarative memory: Priming[††] Language	Declarative memory: Semantic memory[†††] (remain stable or improve)

*Ability to process information speedily to execute cognitive tasks efficiently in a limited period of time.
**Ability to maintain and manipulate a critical, yet limited, amount of information with several options, and consequences.
***Ability to consciously remember, recognize, or recollect past experiences.
****Ability to plan, retain, and retrieve an intention as planned in the future.
[†] Ability to perform a routine daily task unconsciously.
[††] Ability to easily identify a stimulus after a previous exposure to a relevant stimulus.
[†††] Explicit storage of knowledge/categorical information, and word meanings.

goals. The mechanisms of integration and controlling of these neural functions are named "executive control." Along with other higher cognitive functions such as anticipation, judgment, planning, and decision-making, executive functions have a close relationship with the prefrontal cortex.[32]

While age-related cognitive changes are common in the elderly, they are not inevitable outcomes of aging, and are not uniform, with some abilities diminishing more rapidly than others.[33] (See Table 1.1.) For example, despite a decline in the attention and processing speed with aging, decision-making and language functions usually remain stable. Even in memory function, ability to perform a routine daily task (the procedural motor skills memory) may often remain unchanged. It is postulated that age-related declines in many cognitive domains may be due to changes of executive control. Along with other higher cognitive functions such as anticipation, judgment, planning, and decision-making, executive functions have a close relationship with the prefrontal cortex.[32] It was shown that white matter changes, atrophy, and certain forms of neurotransmitter depletion in frontal lobes[34] may lead to executive dysfunctions.

Human Diversity: Inter- and Intra-Individual Variability in Cognitive Abilities

One of the most well-known landmarks in downtown Chicago is a huge 50-foot, 162 ton sculpture with a totally abstract shape resembling a bird, a horse, or a woman. This masterpiece was designed by Picasso and donated by him to the people of Chicago, and named in his honor the "Chicago Picasso" or "Picasso" (Figure 1.3). One interesting fact about this famous sculpture is that Picasso completed a maquette of the sculpture in 1965 and approved the final model in 1966, when he was eighty-five years old.

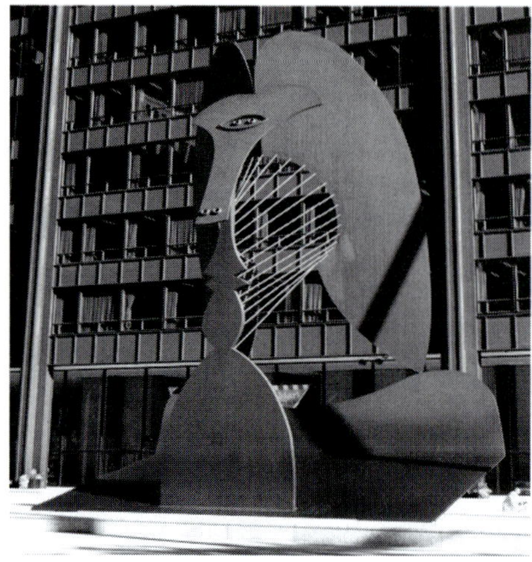

Figure 1.3 "Chicago Picasso," a landmark in downtown Chicago, was designed by Pablo Picasso at age eighty-five years.
(Photo courtesy of L. Hachinski.)

There are several other examples throughout history, like the Picasso sculpture, where older adults were able to retain their mental abilities and perform well or even better than younger ones. It seems that while aging is an undeniable part of life, cognitive decline is not an inevitable part and that significant inter-individual variability can be observed in mental abilities. This rich diversity in human behavior and cognitive abilities in aging has opened a new window to clinical and neuro-functional imaging research in the field of aging and cognition.[35,36,37] A range of factors from genetic background to socioeconomic and educational status, probably contribute to inter-individual variability. Interestingly, functional imaging studies provide insight into the different patterns of brain activity, and more efficient use of brain networks and/or greater ability to recruit alternative networks in the elderly with better cognitive performance.[35,37]

It has also been demonstrated that there are age-dependent intra-individual inconsistencies in performance in neurocognitive tests, such as reaction times[38] that may change from both moment to moment and from day to day.[39] This intra-individual variability has also a stable pattern across time and occasion, which means individuals with greater levels of inconsistency may have more inconsistency at other tasks and testing occasions.[40,41] Moreover, it may affect long-term cognitive outcomes.[42] It is postulated that aging may be associated with a decrease in the stability of executive control over time, which in turn, may lead to inter-individual variability.[43,44]

Finally, it is also important to know the stability of individual differences in cognitive ability across the life course. In one important cohort study, the Lothian Birth Cohort, the intelligence of almost every child born in 1921 and 1936 attending school in Scotland in the month of June in those years was evaluated. The reassessment of these individuals' cognitive ability at age ninety years, showed moderately high stability from childhood to old-old age.[45] Therefore, in definition, classification, and interpretation of neuropsychiatric tests, the importance of intra-individual inconsistencies should always be considered by clinicians and researchers.

Differences in Brain Structures of Men and Women

The lifetime prevalence rates, symptoms and final outcomes of several neuropsychiatric disorders vary significantly between the sexes.[46,47] Understanding the neuroanatomical and functional differences between the male and female brains may help to elucidate the reasons for gender-specific differences among diseases. A combination of genetic,[48,49] steroid hormones, immune systems,[50] and postnatal factors can lead to sex differences in brain structure.[51] Interestingly, these differences emerge as early as the prenatal period and continue throughout the lifespan.

The brain size of male neonates is approximately 6 percent larger than those of female.[52] A result of a recent meta-analysis showed that differences in overall brain volumes are sustained between males and females from newborns to individuals over eighty years old. The most striking differences were reported in limbic and language systems. While in men, volume increases and higher densities were mostly reported in bilateral limbic areas, left posterior cingulate gyrus, and to the left side of the limbic system respectively, larger volumes in females were more frequently seen in special areas in the right hemisphere related to language and to several limbic structures such as the right insular cortex and anterior cingulate gyrus.[53] In addition, women exhibited greater total percentage brain volume loss than men during midlife. While the more extensive volume reduction occurs on the lateral edge of women's brains, it is more significant in midline structures in men.[54] Interestingly, although the results of studies regarding cerebral blood flow in men and women vary, several researchers have shown a higher (about 11 percent or 5 ml/100 g/min) global blood flow in women than in men.[30,55–57].

Finally cognitive performances vary between men and women. Women often show a relatively better performance in working memory,[58] episodic memory, and verbal fluency tasks,[59] whereas men are better in spatial tasks and mathematical problem solving.[60]

Alzheimer-Prone Bias in the Definition and Classification of Dementia

Although in the early twentieth century, vascular disease with hardening of arteries was considered as the main culprit for dementia, several factors have contributed to an "Alzheimerization" bias in favor of neurodegenerative causes of dementia (Figure 1.4).

First and foremost, considering "memory loss" as a core symptom for diagnosis of dementia is the leading source of bias in dementia research. Since cognitive impairment of vascular origin is a heterogeneous group of brain disorders, it may present with a range of cognitive dysfunctions, and in particular, executive dysfunctions. Such definition can dramatically exclude cases of vascular cognitive impairment. Secondly, ideal population-based studies regarding dementia, and in particular cognitive impairment associated with vascular diseases, are scant,[61] and it is not possible to compare many studies since their inclusion criteria and definition for vascular cognitive impairment are not usually interchangeable.[62,63] Therefore, the reported prevalence of vascular cognitive impairment may significantly vary in population-based studies.[62] Different methods of study design and follow up in epidemiological studies on one hand, and restrictive inclusion criteria for vascular cognitive impairment and finally sensitivity and specificity of applied clinical criteria on the other hand, have led to underestimation of the actual rate of vascular origins in dementia studies.[64–66] In addition, the higher rate of death of dementia with

Source of Bias toward AD		Suggestive soloution to decrease the bias		
Rule out Pathological method for Vascular diagnosis	AD	VCI	Revised pathological criteria	Lesser importance
Clinic based studies	AD	VCI	Population based studies	
MMSE	AD	VCI	MoCA and reaction time, development of new tests	Greater importance
Memory based definition of dementia	AD	VCI	Assessment of executive function	
AD: Alzheimer's Disease; VCI: Vascular Cognitive Impairment; MMSE: Mini Mental State Examination; MoCA: Montreal Cognitive Assessment.				

Figure 1.4 Source of bias toward Alzheimerization and suggestive solution to decrease the bias. AD: Alzheimer Disease; VCI: Vascular Cognitive Impairment; MMSE: Mini Mental State Examination; MoCA: Montreal Cognitive Assessment.

cerebrovascular diseases, probably due to comorbid coronary artery diseases, in comparison to Alzheimer disease[67] can also be another reason for the perceived lower prevalence of the former.

Moreover, most epidemiological and clinical studies use the mini mental state examination (MMSE) for screening.[68] This instrument is sensitive to memory impairment, the hallmark of Alzheimer disease, but insensitive to impairments of executive function[69] that may be a hallmark of cerebrovascular disease. Consequently, since executive dysfunction goes undetected, many cases of cognitive impairment due to vascular disease are excluded and ignored (Figure 1.5). The same source of bias can be also observed in many epidemiological studies, where reaction time, as a symptom due to vascular lesions in the frontal lobes or cortico-basal ganglionic–thalamic circuits[70] has not been evaluated. It is important to know that there are still no accurate neuropsychological tests to diagnose vascular cognitive impairment and differentiate it from other common causes of neurodegenerative dementia, largely in part because all major dementias have a vascular component, ranging from 60 percent in frontotemporal dementia to 80 percent in Alzheimer disease.[71]

Although the Montreal Cognitive Assessment (MoCA) has been increasingly used for detecting post-stroke cognitive impairment, even MoCA cannot thoroughly assess all cognitive domains affected following stroke.[72] This is a major obstacle to an accurate clinical diagnosis and consequently preventive strategies and new research. Therefore, it is quite important to develop common standards to identify subjects with cognitive impairment, particularly in the early stages, and especially those with vascular origins of dementia.[73]

The other contributing factor was the creation of Alzheimer centers. Most of these run memory clinics. Patients going to memory clinics, if they have memory impairment not due to depression, are likely to have Alzheimer disease, thus creating a tremendous ascertainment bias in favor of those who have Alzheimer pathology in their brains. In addition, many

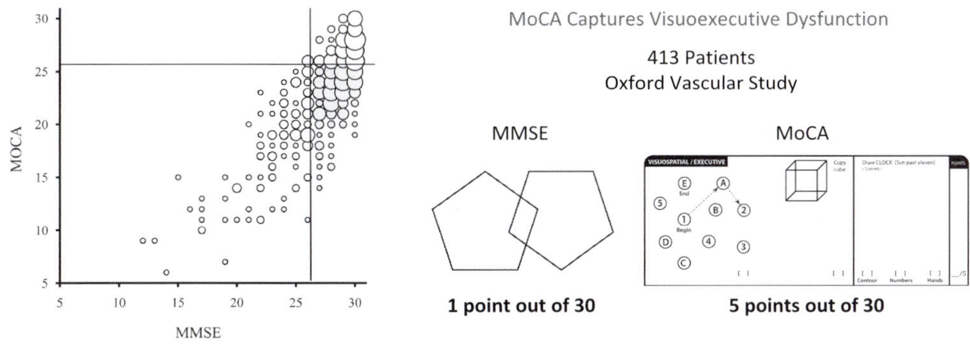

Figure 1.5 Underestimation of cognitive impairment by MMSE vs. MoCA in patients with stroke and TIA. Pendlebury ST, Cuthbertson FC, Welch SJV, Mehta Z, Rothwell PM. Underestimation of cognitive impairment by Mini-Mental State Examination versus the Montreal Cognitive Assessment in patients with transient ischemic attack and stroke: a population-based study. *Stroke: A Journal of Cerebral Circulation*. 2010;41(6):1290–1293.

cases with stroke are followed in stroke outpatient clinics or stroke centers. As a result, non-population-based memory clinic studies can easily underestimate this large group of patients. Physicians also have a tendency to ignore vascular cognitive impairment in their daily practice.

While early signs of memory impairment in the elderly due to medial temporal lobe lesions may easily lead to diagnosis of possible Alzheimer disease, the different localization of vascular pathology and more heterogeneous clinical manifestations, particularly in executive function,[74,75] may unintentionally be ignored and lead to this false, yet common belief that vascular cognitive impairment is an uncommon medical condition. In addition, in the preclinical phases of dementia due to Alzheimer or vascular diseases, similar patterns of cognitive deficits may be observed,[76,77] partially explained by the atrophy in the medial part of the temporal lobe in both conditions.[78] It is also important to know that the underlying pathologies in the majority of community-based demented individuals are a combination between Alzheimer disease and vascular changes.[79] This pattern differs in clinic-based cohorts where atypical forms of dementia and uncommon types such as Lewy body dementia can be seen more frequently,[80] which is another source of bias for under-estimation of vascular pathology. In addition, most of the clinical pathological reports of patients are from Alzheimer centers, and they do not take into account that about one-fifth of patients initially diagnosed with having Alzheimer disease do not progress.[81] Typically, clinical pathological studies only include those subjects who deteriorate and die. However, if one adds the denominator of those who do not progress, the accuracy rates of the initial diagnosis of Alzheimer disease is much less than reported in the literature.

The diagnosis of pure Alzheimer disease is accurate only 38 percent of the time,[81] a proportion that has not significantly improved with sophisticated PET brain imaging and cerebrospinal fluid (CSF) biomarkers (only 4 pure Alzheimer disease cases out of a consecutive series of the first 22 presumed Alzheimer disease).[71]

Finally, despite the fact that pathological findings are the gold standard for the majority of diseases, neuropathological criteria for diagnosis of vascular dementia are still a matter of debate,[82,83] and pathological diagnosis of dementia due to vascular disease is based on the exclusion of other causes of dementia (default diagnosis). While such approach seems to be rational due to the high rate of vascular pathology in the elderly, this type of definition may also cause an underestimation of the prevalence of pure/mixed type of vascular cognitive impairment.

The Resurgence of Cerebrovascular Disease

The rise of Alzheimer disease made things simple again. Alzheimer disease became near synonymous with dementia as "atherosclerosis" of the brain arteries had been. However, with the advent of brain imaging, computed axial tomography (CAT) scanning, and Magnetic Resonance Imaging (MRI) in the 1980s and 1990s, vascular disease regained a part in the diagnostic repertoire again, through the demonstration of white matter changes in cognitively impaired patients.

These white matter changes were immediately attributed with profligate ease to "Binswanger disease," "vascular encephalopathy," "microvascular disease," and "chronic ischemia." The same facile thinking used to explain deterioration by chronic ischemia affecting grey matter was now applied to white matter with no more evidence for the latter than the former. It was suggested that the white matter changes were non-specific and until we sorted out the multiple etiologies it was best to use a descriptive term such as "leukoaraiosis," meaning white matter rarefication.[84] It is also observed that while white matter changes are a prevalent finding among patients suffering from vascular cognitive impairment,[85] these findings can also be frequently seen in asymptomatic elderly patients.[86] In symptomatic individuals, besides cognitive problems and especially executive dysfunction, symptoms include depression,[87,88] and movement disorders such as parkinsonism,[89–91] which may be explained by the disruption in pre-frontal sub-cortical circuits due to white matter lesions or stroke.[92–94]

The Vascular Cognitive Impairment Approach

It was slowly realized that while Alzheimer disease is often progressive and fatal, vascular lesions are not necessarily progressive and that the cognitive impairment spans a whole spectrum between mild cognitive impairment to dementia and hence the term "vascular cognitive impairment" was suggested to describe the whole range of any cognitive impairment due to or associated with vascular disease.[95,96] To date, this remains the only treatable and preventable component. It was also discovered that for each clinical stroke there are probably five so-called silent strokes where upon closer examination, patients exhibit subtle neurological signs and cognitive impairment.[97]

It was also suggested that if we are to be successful, prevention should start early, perhaps at the "brain at risk stage" when there are no clinical manifestations, but risk factors are present to try to prevent or delay subsequent strokes and/or cognitive impairment.[98] For example, it was clearly shown that chronic hypertension can affect small end arteries located in the brainstem and the center of the brain. The medial and basal portions of the brain and brainstem are supplied by relatively short arteries penetrating the brain in the basal dorsal direction. Since these arteries arise from large basal trunks, the gradation between arterial and capillary pressure occurs over a relatively short distance, requiring the arteries to withstand high pressure. Functionally, arteries in the upper brainstem and diencephalon (centrecephalon) are end arteries without substantial collateral supply from adjacent vessels. Therefore, occlusion of a centrecephalon artery usually leads to a small infarct, because it supplies a limited cylinder of tissue (Figure 1.6).[99] Due to

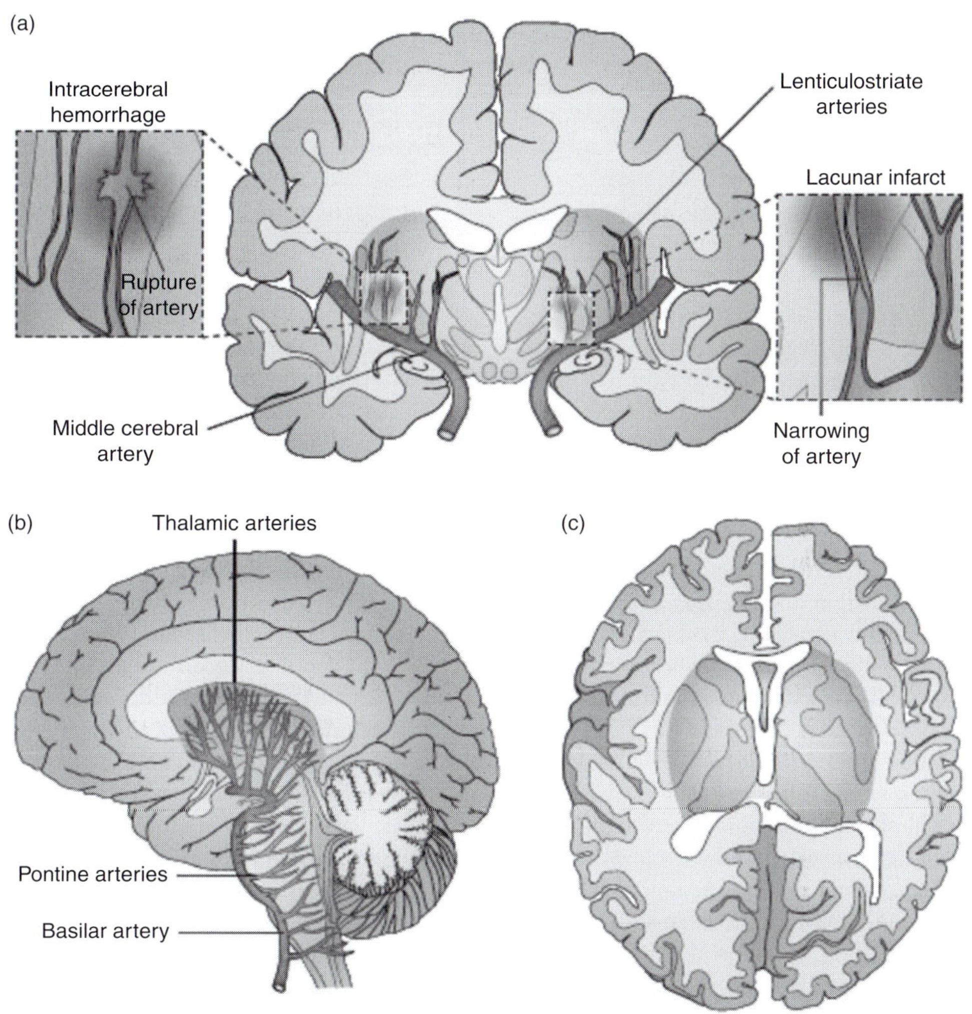

Figure 1.6 The role of end arteries in the pathophysiology of lacunar infarcts and intracerebral hemorrhages. Sörös P, Whitehead S, Spence JD, Hachinski V. Antihypertensive treatment can prevent stroke and cognitive decline. Nat Rev Neurol. 2013;9:174–178.

significant correlation between cognitive decline and stroke in patients with and without Alzheimer disease pathology, it seems that in patients of all ages, not treating hypertension is a missed opportunity to prevent some of the most prevalent brain diseases.[99]

Epidemiology of Aging-Associated Cognitive Changes and Vascular Cognitive Impairment

Based on a recent report from the WHO (www.who.int/ageing/publications/global_health), for the first time in the history of mankind, it was predicted that the number of people aged sixty-five or older will outnumber children under age five (Figure 1.7). This report also indicates that the population of the elderly, aged sixty-five years and over, was 524 million in

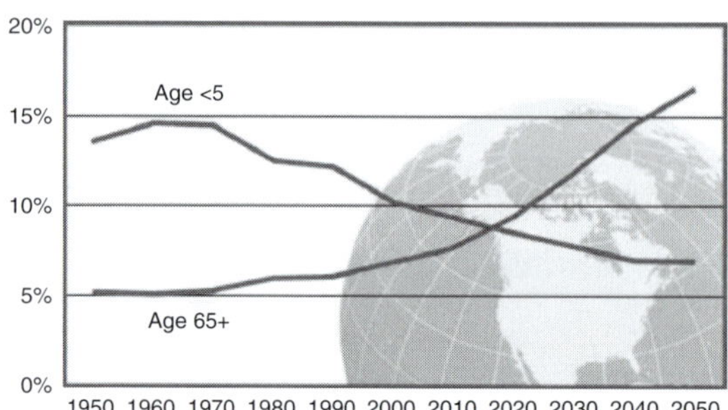

Figure 1.7 Young children and older people as a percentage of global population: 1950–2050. Adapted from World Population Prospects: The 2010 Revision, by United Nations, Department of Economic and Social Affairs, Population Division, © 2011 United Nations. Reprinted with the permission of the United Nations.

2010 and will reach 1.5 billion in 2050. A higher rate of age-related diseases, such as dementia, can therefore be expected worldwide.[100] However, the majority of the elderly do not show significant cognitive decline with functional impairments and are able to live independently. In other words, while cognitive abilities are vulnerable to the processes of aging, patterns, severity, and cognitive domains of age-associated changes of cognitive abilities vary significantly. In addition, cognitive changes can be under the influence of inter- and intra-individual variability. Therefore, it is of paramount importance for clinicians to differentiate cognitive changes in advanced age from clinical signs of dementia, and not assume that any changes in the cognition of the elderly is a symptom of dementia.

The prevalence of stroke and dementia varies significantly worldwide. Stroke and dementia occur roughly with the same frequency, but about a decade apart (Figure 1.8).[101] Stroke incidence is falling in developed countries and rising in middle- and low-income countries (Figure 1.9).[102,103] It is tempting to conclude that the rise in the incidence of stroke in the middle- and low-incomes countries reflects westernization and the growth of cities, where to get fast food is easy, but to get exercise is hard. The fact that the incidence has changed so dramatically over the last few decades suggests that genes may play only a modest role at the population level and that whatever factors have caused such significant rise in low- and middle-income countries and fall in high-income countries are modifiable.

A similar pattern has been shown in dementia incidence, which is rising globally,[104] but tending to fall in some developed countries.[105] Based on a recent meta-analysis, it is estimated that 35.6 million people suffered from dementia worldwide in 2010, more than a half living in low- or middle-income countries.[106] One cross-sectional survey of 14,960 individuals in seven low- or middle-income countries showed that the DSM–IV criteria may significantly underestimate the true prevalence of dementia.[107] Therefore, it is even more difficult to estimate the exact rate of dementia in such countries. The estimation of the accurate rate of vascular cognitive impairment is even more difficult. The prevalence of dementia continuously increases with age, ranging from 2–3 percent among those aged 70–75 years to 20–25 percent among those aged 85 years or more.[108] Although a similar scenario can be expected in vascular cognitive impairment,[109] its prevalence was not equal in the world.[110,111] For example, while a higher prevalence of vascular cognitive impairment was reported in Japan,[112] since 1990, Alzheimer disease has become more common in China.[113] Valid data about middle-eastern countries are scant.

The prevalence of dementia after stroke also varied in different studies, ranging from 6 percent to 32 percent, based on the time and method of evaluation. The result of one meta-analysis showed that 10 percent of patients had dementia before first stroke, and about 10 percent developed new dementia soon after the first stroke at the rate which increased to

(a)

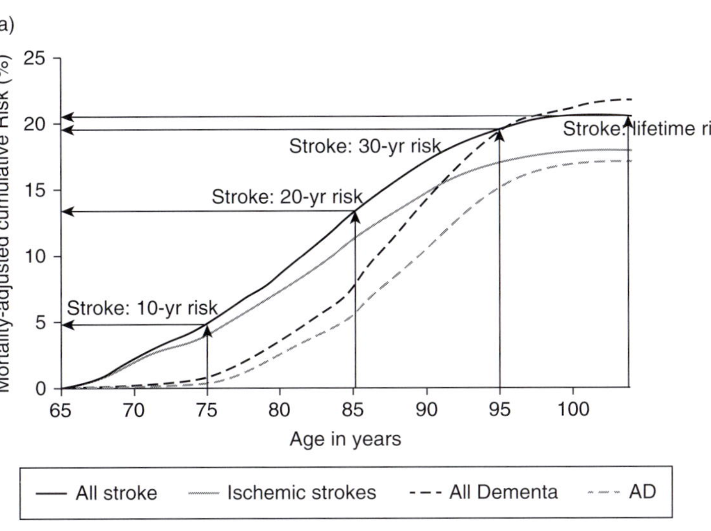

Figure 1.8 The lifetime risk of stroke and dementia in women and men 65 years of age. Seshadri S, Beiser A, Kelly-Hayes M, et al. The lifetime risk of stroke: estimates from the Framingham Study. *Stroke.* 2006;37:345–350.

(b)

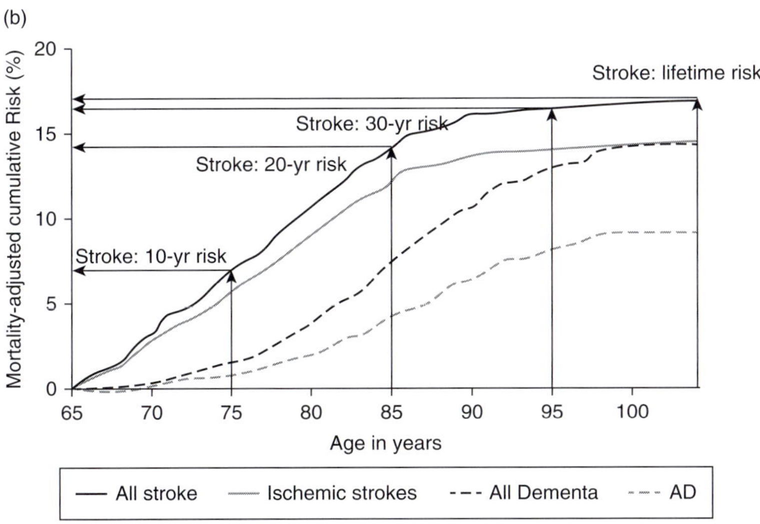

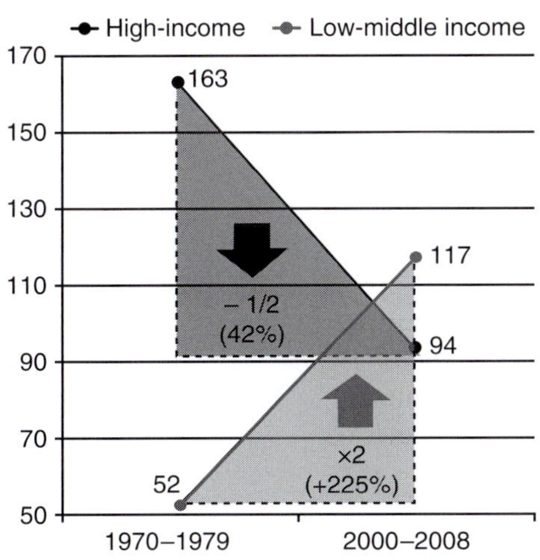

Figure 1.9 Age-adjusted stroke incidence rate per 100,000 persons in high- vs. low-middle income countries. Reproduced with permission from Elsevier from: Feigin VL, Lawes CM, Bennett DA, Barker-Collo SL, Parag V. Worldwide stroke incidence and early case fatality reported in 56 population based studies: a systematic review. *The Lancet Neurology.* 2009;8(4):355–369.

one-third after stroke recurrence.[114] It was also shown that slope of cognitive decline may become steeper after stroke.[115] Moreover, stroke doubles the likelihood of developing dementias.[116] Recently, studies have shown a decrease in the incidence of stroke at a whole-population level, followed a few years later by a decline in the incidence of dementia, suggesting that preventing stroke may also prevent some dementias (Figure 1.10).[117]

A New Era Begins

Vascular lesions, Alzheimer lesions, and Lewy bodies are common in elderly individuals; however, it is multiple pathologies that increase the risk of developing cognitive impairment.[79] In a large autopsy series of 6,205 patients, it was established that all major dementias have a vascular component, ranging from 60 percent frontotemporal dementias to 80 percent in Alzheimer disease(Figure 1.11).[71] It seems that having a vascular component can double the chance that neurodegenerative pathologies will result in dementia. In fact, the largest component of cognitive impairment can be explained by vascular and/or

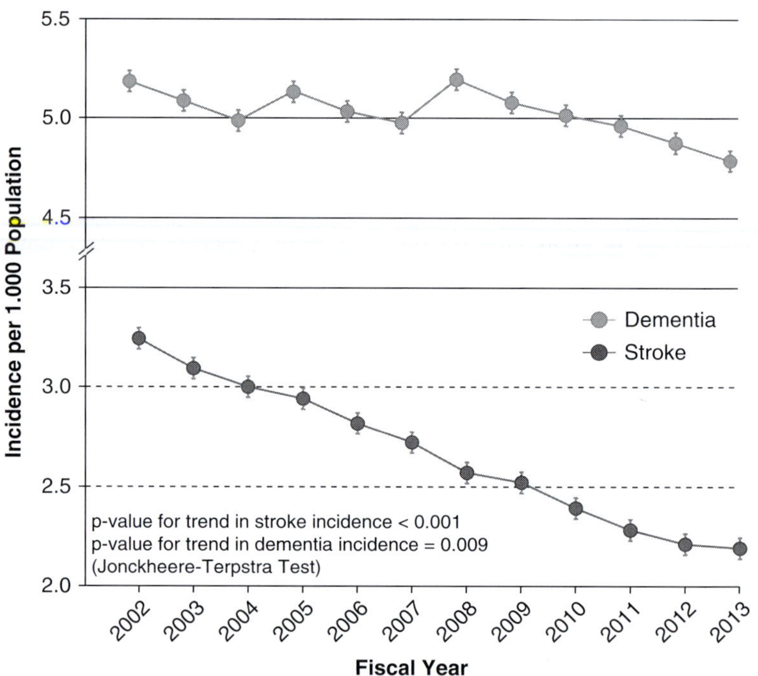

Figure 1.10 Decreasing incidence of dementia in developed countries. Sposato LA, Kapral MK, Fang J, et al. Declining incidence of stroke and dementia: coincidence or prevention opportunity? *JAMA Neurology.* 2015;72(12):1529–1531.

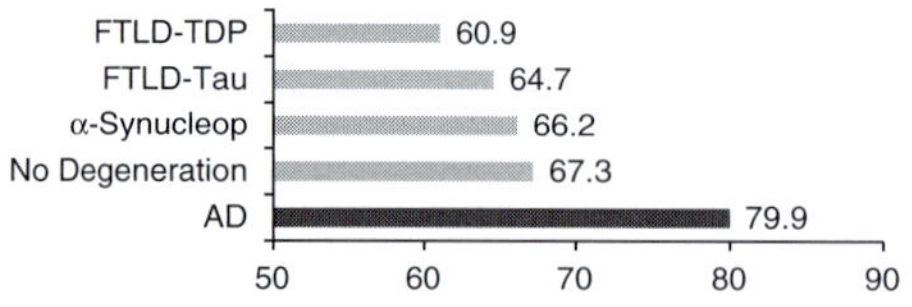

Figure 1.11 Prevalence of vascular pathology (percent) in autopsy-confirmed neurodegenerative disease of 6205 cases. Toledo, J. B., Arnold, S. E., Raible, K., et al. Contribution of cerebrovascular disease in autopsy confirmed neurodegenerative disease cases in the National Alzheimer's Coordinating Centre. Brain. 2013;136(Pt 9):2697–2706.

Table 1.2 Main proposed common risk and protective factors for stroke and dementia. Modified from Solomon et al[120]

Non-Modifiable		Modifiable
Risk factors	Risk factors	Protective factors
Advanced age	Cerebrovascular disease / Stroke	High education
Genetic factors (Apo E4)	Cardiovascular diseases	Physical activity
Family history	Hypertensions	Antihypertensive
	Hypercholesterolemia	Statins
	Obesity	Active lifestyle
	Diabetes	Healthy diet*
	Atrial fibrillation	Anticoagulant medications*
	Smoking	
	Homocysteinemia	
	Stress	
	Depression	

*Added

Alzheimer disease. This suggests that we may discover additional pathologies and also protective features. The good news is that it is now possible to study many of these pathological processes "in vivo," such as vascular disease and amyloid and tau protein deposition and inflammation by positron emission tomography and an increasing number of bio and genetic markers.[118]

The fact that the incidence is falling where stroke has declined also suggests that controlling risk factors may account partially for this, since the risk factors and enhancing factors for stroke and dementia are the same,[119,120] (Table 1.2). This trend can be partially explained by common use of antihypertensive antidyslipidaemic medications and a decrement in smoking rate;[119] however, the increased prevalence of obesity and sedentary lifestyle may lead to another epidemiological shift toward cerebrovascular diseases.[121] Not surprisingly, while at present, despite all Alzheimerization bias, vascular disease is considered the second-most-important reason for cognitive impairment, and it may become the most common form of dementia in the elderly.[92] In other words, cases with pathological findings of pure Alzheimer disease can be quite asymptomatic throughout life. Therefore, it is also possible that vascular disease not only leads to vascular cognitive impairments, but also expresses other neurodegenerative types of dementia such as Alzheimer disease.[79,119,122] One possible explanation can be an increase in A-β generation or decrease clearance[123] even in patients without a new ischemic lesion.[124–126] This may also raise one major question: Can vascular pathology enhance the formation of Alzheimer disease lesions, or can it merely add to the severity of clinical symptoms?[122]

These considerations may change our traditional dichotomy classification and the black and white bordering definition of dementia to "senile" versus "pre-senile" and "Alzheimer" versus "vascular" and perhaps lead to a broader, unbiased definition of dementia. This may lead to the beginning, or at least a fair acknowledgment, of a new era in a definition and classification of cognitive impairment that is "treatable and potentially preventable."

References

1. Hachinski VC, Lassen NA, Marshall J. Multi-infarct dementia: a cause of mental deterioration in the elderly. *Lancet* 1974;2:207–210.

2. McKhann G, Drachman D, Folstein M, Katzman R, Price D, Stadlan EM. Clinical diagnosis of Alzheimer's disease: Report of the NINCDS-ADRDA Work Group* under the auspices of Department of Health and Human Services Task Force on Alzheimer's Disease. *Neurol.* 1983;**34**:939–939.

3. Paulson OB. Blood-brain barrier, brain metabolism and cerebral blood flow. *Eur Neuropsychopharmacol: J Eur Coll Neuropsychopharmacol.* 2002;**12**:495–501.

4. Gilkes CE, Whitfield PC. Intracranial pressure and cerebral blood flow: a pathophysiological and clinical perspective. *Surg.* 2009;**27**:139–134.

5. Ito H, Kanno I, Fukuda H. Human cerebral circulation: positron emission tomography studies. *Ann Nucl Med.* 2009;**19**(2):65-74.

6. Akers D, Sherbondy A, Mackenzie R, Dougherty R, Wandell B. Exploration of the brain's white matter pathways with dynamic queries. In: IEEE Visualization 2004 IEEE Comput. Soc. 2003; 377–384.

7. Zhang K, Sejnowski TJ. A universal scaling law between gray matter and white matter of cerebral cortex. *Proc Natl Acad Sci United States Am.* 2000;**97**:5621–5626.

8. Guan T, Kong J. Functional regeneration of the brain: white matter matters. *Neural Regen Res.* 2015;**10**:355–356.

9. Hinman JD, Abraham CR. What's behind the decline? The role of white matter in brain aging. *Neurochem Res.* 2007;**32**:2023–2031.

10. Reich T, Rusinek H. Cerebral cortical and white matter reactivity to carbon dioxide. *Stroke.* 1989;**20**:453–357.

11. Ito H, Kanno I, Fukuda H. Human cerebral circulation: positron emission tomography studies. *Ann Nucl Med.* 2005;**19**:65–74.

12. Matsushita K, Kuriyama Y, Nagatsuka K, Nakamura M, Sawada T, Omae T. Periventricular white matter lucency and cerebral blood flow autoregulation in hypertensive patients. *Hypertens.* 1994;**23**:565–8.

13. Prins ND, van Dijk EJ, den Heijer T, et al. Cerebral white matter lesions and the risk of dementia. *Arch Neurol.* 2004;**61**:1531–1534.

14. Ballabh P, Braun A, Nedergaard M. The blood-brain barrier: an overview: structure, regulation, and clinical implications. *Neurobiol Dis.* 2004;**16**:1–13.

15. Hawkins BT, Davis TP. The blood-brain barrier/neurovascular unit in health and disease. *Pharmacol Rev.* 2005;**57**: 173–185.

16. Butt AM, Jones HC, Abbott NJ. Electrical resistance across the blood-brain barrier in anaesthetized rats: a developmental study. *J Physiol.* 1990;**429**:47–62.

17. Kniesel U, Wolburg H. Tight junctions of the blood-brain barrier. *Cell Mol Neurobiol.* 2000;**20**:57–76.

18. Abbott NJ. Astrocyte-endothelial interactions and blood-brain barrier permeability. *J Anat.* 2002;**200**(6):629-638.

19. Bell RD, Winkler EA, Sagare AP, et al. Pericytes control key neurovascular functions and neuronal phenotype in the adult brain and during brain aging. *Neuron.* 2010;**68**:409–427.

20. McCaffrey G, Davis TP. Physiology and pathophysiology of the blood-brain barrier: P-glycoprotein and occludin trafficking as therapeutic targets to optimize central nervous system drug delivery. *J Investig Med : Off Publ Am Fed Clin Res.* 2012;**60**:1131–1140.

21. Iliff JJ, Wang M, Liao Y, et al. A paravascular pathway facilitates CSF flow through the brain parenchyma and the clearance of interstitial solutes, including amyloid β. *Sci Transl Med.* 2012;4.

22. Iliff JJ, Nedergaard M. Is there a cerebral lymphatic system? *Stroke*. 2013;**44**: S93–S95.

23. Kirkness CJ. Cerebral blood flow monitoring in clinical practice. *AACN Clin issues*. 2005 **16**:476–487.

24. Willie CK, Tzeng Y-C, Fisher JA, Ainslie PN. Integrative regulation of human brain blood flow. *J Physiol*. 2014;**592**:841–859.

25. Elias MF, D'Agostino RB, Elias PK, Wolf PA. Neuropsychological test performance, cognitive functioning, blood pressure, and age: the Framingham Heart Study. *Exp Aging Res*. 1995;**21**:369–391.

26. Waldemar G, Hasselbalch SG, Andersen AR, et al. 99mTc-d,l-HMPAO and SPECT of the brain in normal aging. *J Cereb Blood Flow Metab : Off J Int Soc Cereb Blood Flow Metab* [Internet]. 1991 May 1 [cited 1991 May 1];**11**:508–521.

27. Marchal G, Rioux P, Petit-Taboué MC, et al. Regional cerebral oxygen consumption, blood flow, and blood volume in healthy human aging. *Arch Neurol*. 1992;**49**:1013–1020.

28. Kashimada A, Machida K, Honda N, et al. Measurement of cerebral blood flow with two-dimensional cine phase-contrast mR imaging: evaluation of normal subjects and patients with vertigo. *Radiat Med*. 1995;**13**:95–102.

29. Buijs PC, Krabbe-Hartkamp MJ, Bakker CJ, et al. Effect of age on cerebral blood flow: measurement with ungated two-dimensional phase-contrast MR angiography in 250 adults. *Radiology*. 1998;**209**:667–674.

30. Parkes LM, Rashid W, Chard DT, Tofts PS. Normal cerebral perfusion measurements using arterial spin labeling: reproducibility, stability, and age and gender effects. *Magn Reson Med*. 2004;**51**:736–743.

31. Shin W, Horowitz S, Ragin A, Chen Y, Walker M, Carroll TJ. Quantitative cerebral perfusion using dynamic susceptibility contrast MRI: evaluation of reproducibility and age- and gender-dependence with fully automatic image postprocessing algorithm. *Magn Reson Med*. 2007;**58**:1232–41.

32. Funahashi S, Andreau JM. Prefrontal cortex and neural mechanisms of executive function. *J Physiol Paris*. 2013;**107**:471–482.

33. Salthouse TA. *Theoretical Perspectives on Cognitive Aging*. New York, NY: Psychology Press; 2015.

34. Buckner RL. Memory and executive function in aging and AD. *Neuron*. 2004;**44**:195–208.

35. Cabeza R, Anderson ND, Locantore JK, McIntosh AR. Aging gracefully: compensatory brain activity in high-performing older adults. *NeuroImage*. 2002;**17**:1394–1402.

36. Kanai R, Rees G. The structural basis of inter-individual differences in human behaviour and cognition. *Nat Rev Neurosci*. 2011;**12**:231–242.

37. Bastin C, Yakushev I, Bahri MA, et al. Cognitive reserve impacts on inter-individual variability in resting-state cerebral metabolism in normal aging. *NeuroImage*. 2012;**63**:713–722.

38. Williams BR, Hultsch DF, Strauss EH, Hunter MA, Tannock R. Inconsistency in reaction time across the life span. *Neuropsychology* [Internet]. 2005 Jan 1 [cited 2005 Jan 1];**19**:88–96.

39. Rabbitt P, Osman P, Moore B, Stollery B. There are stable individual differences in performance variability, both from moment to moment and from day to day. *Q J Exp Psychol Hum Exp Psychol*. 2001;**54**:981–1003.

40. Rabbitt P, Osman P, Moore B, Stollery B. There are stable individual differences in performance variability, both from moment to moment and from day to day. *Q J Exp Psychol Sect*. 2001;**54**:981–1003.

41. Fuentes K, Hunter MA, Strauss E, Hultsch DF. Intraindividual variability in cognitive performance in persons with chronic fatigue syndrome. *Clin Neuropsychol*. 2001;**15**:210–227.

42. Bielak AAM, Hultsch DF, Strauss E, Macdonald SWS, Hunter MA. Intraindividual variability in reaction time predicts cognitive outcomes 5 years later. *Neuropsychology.* 2010;**24**:731–741.

43. West R, Murphy KJ, Armilio ML, Craik FIM, Stuss DT. Lapses of intention and performance variability reveal age-related increases in fluctuations of executive control. *Brain Cogn.* 2002;**49**:402–419.

44. Jackson JD, Balota DA, Duchek JM, Head D. White matter integrity and reaction time intraindividual variability in healthy aging and early-stage Alzheimer disease. *Neuropsychologia.* 2012;**50**:357–366.

45. Deary IJ, Pattie A, Starr JM. The stability of intelligence from age 11 to age 90 years: the Lothian birth cohort of 1921. *Psychol Sci.* 2013;**24**:2361–2368.

46. Gur RC, Turetsky BI, Matsui M, et al. Sex differences in brain gray and white matter in healthy young adults: correlations with cognitive performance. *J Neurosci : Off J Soc Neurosci.* 1999;**19**:4065–4072.

47. Paus T. Sex differences in the human brain: a developmental perspective. *Prog Brain Res.* 2009 ;**186**:13–28.

48. Kang HJ, Kawasawa YI, Cheng F, et al. Spatio-temporal transcriptome of the human brain. *Nature.* 2011;**478**:483–489.

49. De Vries GJ, Rissman EF, Simerly RB, et al. A model system for study of sex chromosome effects on sexually dimorphic neural and behavioral traits. *J Neurosci : Off J Soc Neurosci.* 2002;**22**:9005–9014.

50. Lenz KM, Nugent BM, Haliyur R, McCarthy MM. Microglia are essential to masculinization of brain and behavior. *J Neurosci : Off J Soc Neurosci.* 2013;**33**:2761–2772.

51. Becker JB, Arnold AP, Berkley KJ, et al. Strategies and methods for research on sex differences in brain and behavior. *Endocrinology.* 2005;**146**:1650–1673.

52. Viveros M-P, Mendrek A, Paus T, et al. A comparative, developmental, and clinical perspective of neurobehavioral sexual dimorphisms. *Front Neurosci.* 2012;**6**:84.

53. Ruigrok ANV, Salimi-Khorshidi G, Lai M-C, et al. A meta-analysis of sex differences in human brain structure. *Neurosci & Biobehav Rev.* 2013;**39**:34–50.

54. Guo JY, Isohanni M, Miettunen J, et al. Brain structural changes in women and men during midlife. *Neurosci Lett.* 2016;**615**:107–112.

55. Gur RC, Gur RE, Obrist WD, Skolnick BE, Reivich M. Age and regional cerebral blood flow at rest and during cognitive activity. *Arch Gen Psychiatry.* 1987;**44**:617–621.

56. Rootwelt K, Dybevold S, Nyberg-Hansen R, Russell D. Measurement of cerebral blood flow with 133Xe inhalation and dynamic single photon emission computer tomography. Normal values. *Scand J Clin Lab Investig Suppl.* 1985;**184**:97–105.

57. Rodriguez G, Warkentin S, Risberg J, Rosadini G. Sex differences in regional cerebral blood flow. *J Cereb Blood Flow Metab : Off J Int Soc Cereb Blood Flow Metab.* 1988;**8**:783–789.

58. Speck O, Ernst T, Braun J, Koch C, Miller E, Chang L. Gender differences in the functional organization of the brain for working memory. *Neuroreport.* 2000;**11**:2581–2585.

59. Herlitz A, Airaksinen E, Nordström E. Sex differences in episodic memory: the impact of verbal and visuospatial ability. *Neuropsychology.* 1999;**13**:590–597.

60. Lewin C, Wolgers G, Herlitz A. Sex differences favoring women in verbal but not in visuospatial episodic memory. *Neuropsychology.* 2001;**15**:165–173.

61. Zaccai J, Ince P, Brayne C. Population-based neuropathological studies of dementia: design, methods and areas of investigation: a systematic review. *BMC Neurol.* 2006;**6**:2.

62. Chui HC, Mack W, Jackson JE, et al. Clinical criteria for the diagnosis of vascular dementia: a multicenter study of comparability and interrater reliability. *Arch Neurol.* 2000;**57**:191–196.

63. Pohjasvaara T, Mantyla R, Ylikoski R, Kaste M, Erkinjuntti T. Comparison of different clinical criteria (DSM-III,

ADDTC, ICD-10, NINDS-AIREN, DSM-IV) for the diagnosis of vascular dementia. *Stroke.* 2000;**31**.

64. Gold G, Giannakopoulos P, Montes-Paixao Júnior C, et al. Sensitivity and specificity of newly proposed clinical criteria for possible vascular dementia. *Neurology.* 1997;**49**:690–694.

65. Knopman DS, Parisi JE, Boeve BF, et al. Vascular dementia in a population-based autopsy study. *Arch Neurol.* 2003;**60**:569–575.

66. Bacchetta J-P, Kövari E, Merlo M, et al. Validation of clinical criteria for possible vascular dementia in the oldest-old. *Neurobiol Aging.* 2007;**28**:579–585.

67. Kalaria RN, Maestre GE, Arizaga R, et al., World Federation of Neurology Dementia Research Group: Alzheimer's disease and vascular dementia in developing countries: prevalence, management, and risk factors. *Lancet Neurol.* 2008;7:812–826.

68. Folstein MF, Folstein SE, McHugh PR. "Mini-mental state": a practical method for grading the cognitive state of patients for the clinician. *J Psychiatr Res.* 1974;**12**:189–198.

69. Pendlebury ST, Cuthbertson FC, Welch SJV, Mehta Z, Rothwell PM. Underestimation of cognitive impairment by mini-mental state examination versus the Montreal cognitive assessment in patients with transient ischemic attack and stroke: a population-based study. *Stroke.* 2009;**41**:1290–1293.

70. Mendez MF, Cherrier MM, Perryman KM. Differences between Alzheimer's disease and vascular dementia on information processing measures. *Brain Cogn.* 1997;**34**:301–310.

71. Toledo JB, Arnold SE, Raible K, et al. Contribution of cerebrovascular disease in autopsy confirmed neurodegenerative disease cases in the National Alzheimer's Coordinating Centre. *Brain : J Neurol.* 2013;**136**:2697–2706.

72. Chan E, Khan S, Oliver R, Gill SK, Werring DJ, Cipolotti L. Underestimation of cognitive impairments by the Montreal Cognitive Assessment (MoCA) in an acute stroke unit population. *J Neurol Sci.* 2014;**343**:176–179.

73. Hachinski V, Iadecola C, Petersen RC, et al. National Institute of Neurological Disorders and Stroke-Canadian Stroke Network vascular cognitive impairment harmonization standards. *Stroke; J Cereb Circ.* 2005;**37**:2220–2241.

74. Sachdev PS, Brodaty H, Valenzuela MJ, et al. The neuropsychological profile of vascular cognitive impairment in stroke and TIA patients. *Neurology.* 2004;**62**:912–919.

75. Nordlund A, Rolstad S, Klang O, Lind K, Hansen S, Wallin A. Cognitive profiles of mild cognitive impairment with and without vascular disease. *Neuropsychology.* 2007;**21**:706–712.

76. Laukka EJ, Jones S, Small BJ, Fratiglioni L, Bäckman L. Similar patterns of cognitive deficits in the preclinical phases of vascular dementia and Alzheimer's disease. *J Int Neuropsychol Soc : JINS.* 2004;**10**:382–391.

77. Bäckman L, Small BJ. Cognitive deficits in preclinical Alzheimer's disease and vascular dementia: patterns of findings from the Kungsholmen Project. *Physiol & Behav.* 2007;**92**:80–86.

78. Firbank MJ, Burton EJ, Barber R, et al. Medial temporal atrophy rather than white matter hyperintensities predict cognitive decline in stroke survivors. *Neurobiol Aging.* 2007;**28**:1664–1669.

79. Schneider JA, Arvanitakis Z, Bang W, Bennett DA. Mixed brain pathologies account for most dementia cases in community-dwelling older persons. *Neurology.* 2007;**69**:2197–2204.

80. Schneider JA, Aggarwal NT, Barnes L, Boyle P, Bennett DA. The neuropathology of older persons with and without dementia from community versus clinic cohorts. *J Alzheimer's Dis.* 2008;**18**:691–701.

81. Bowler JV, Munoz DG, Merskey H, Hachinski V. Fallacies in the pathological confirmation of the diagnosis of Alzheimer's disease. *J Neurol Neurosurgery, Psychiatry.* 1998;**64**:18–24.

82. Pantoni L, Palumbo V, Sarti C. Pathological lesions in vascular dementia. *Ann New York Acad Sci.* 2002;**977**:279–291.

83. Grinberg LT, Heinsen H. Toward a pathological definition of vascular dementia. *J Neurol Sci.* 2010;**299**:136–138.

84. Hachinski VC, Potter P, Merskey H. Leuko-araiosis: an ancient term for a new problem. *Can J Neurol Sci Le J Can des Sci Neurol.* 1986;**13**:533–534.

85. Pantoni L. Cerebral small vessel disease: from pathogenesis and clinical characteristics to therapeutic challenges. *Lancet Neurol.* 2010;**9**:689–701.

86. Launer LJ, Berger K, Breteler MMB, et al. Regional variability in the prevalence of cerebral white matter lesions: an MRI study in 9 European countries (CASCADE). *Neuroepidemiology.* 2006;**26**:23–29.

87. Alexopoulos GS, Meyers BS, Young RC, Campbell S, Silbersweig D, Charlson M. "Vascular depression" hypothesis. *Arch Gen Psychiatry.* 1997;**54**:915–922.

88. Taylor WD, Aizenstein HJ, Alexopoulos GS. The vascular depression hypothesis: mechanisms linking vascular disease with depression. *Mol Psychiatry.* 2013;**18**:963–974.

89. Bansil S, Prakash N, Kaye J, et al. Movement disorders after stroke in adults: a review. *Tremor Other hyperkinetic Movements.* 2012;**2**.

90. Van der Holst HM, van Uden IWM, Tuladhar AM, et al. Cerebral small vessel disease and incident parkinsonism: The RUN DMC study. *Neurology.* 2015;**85**:1569–1577.

91. Luca CC, Rundek T. Parkinsonism, Small vessel disease, and white matter disease: is there a link? *Neurology.* 2015;**85**:1532–1533.

92. Román GC. Vascular dementia may be the most common form of dementia in the elderly. *J Neurol Sci.* 2002;**203**–204:7–10.

93. Román GC, Royall DR. Executive control function: a rational basis for the diagnosis of vascular dementia. *Alzheimer Dis & Assoc Disord.* 1999;**13**.

94. Pohjasvaara T, Leskelä M, Vataja R, et al. Post-stroke depression, executive dysfunction and functional outcome. *Eur J Neurol.* 2002;**9**:269–275.

95. Hachinski VC, Bowler JV. Vascular dementia. *Neurology.* 1993;**43**:2159–2160; author reply 2160–1.

96. Hachinski V. Vascular dementia: a radical redefinition. *Dement.* 1994;**5**:130–132.

97. Vermeer SE, Longstreth WT, Koudstaal PJ. Silent brain infarcts: a systematic review. *Lancet Neurol.* 2007;**6**:611–619.

98. Hachinski V. Preventable senility: a call for action against the vascular dementias. *Lancet.* 1992;**340**:645–648.

99. Sörös P, Whitehead S, Spence JD, Hachinski V. Antihypertensive treatment can prevent stroke and cognitive decline. *Nat Rev Neurol.* 2013;**9**:174–178.

100. Brookmeyer R, Johnson E, Ziegler-Graham K, Arrighi HM. Forecasting the global burden of Alzheimer's disease. *Alzheimer's & Dement : J Alzheimer's Assoc.* 2007;**3**:186–191.

101. Seshadri S, Beiser A, Kelly-Hayes M, et al. The lifetime risk of stroke: estimates from the Framingham Study. *Stroke.* 2006;**37**:345–350.

102. Feigin VL, Lawes CMM, Bennett DA, Barker-Collo SL, Parag V. Worldwide stroke incidence and early case fatality reported in 56 population-based studies: a systematic review. *Lancet Neurol.* 2009;**8**:355–369.

103. Azarpazhooh MR, Etemadi MM, Donnan GA, et al. 2010. Excessive incidence of stroke in Iran: evidence from the Mashhad Stroke Incidence Study (MSIS), a population-based study of stroke in the Middle East. *Stroke.* 2010 Jan 19;**41**: e3–e10.

104. Alzheimer's Association A. 2013 Alzheimer's disease facts and figures. *Alzheimer's & Dement.* 2012;**9**:208–245.

105. Matthews FE, Arthur A, Barnes LE, et al., Medical Research Council Cognitive Function and Ageing Collaboration: a two-decade comparison of prevalence of dementia in individuals aged 65 years and

older from three geographical areas of England: results of the Cognitive Function and Ageing Study I and II. *Lancet*. 2013;**382**:1405–1412.

106. Prince M, Bryce R, Albanese E, Wimo A, Ribeiro W, Ferri CP. The global prevalence of dementia: a systematic review and metaanalysis. *Alzheimer's & Dement: J Alzheimer's Assoc*. 2013;**9**:63–75.e2.

107. Rodriguez JJL, Ferri CP, Acosta D, et al. Prevalence of dementia in Latin America, India, and China: a population-based cross-sectional survey. *Lancet*. 2007;**372**:464–474.

108. Ferri CP, Prince M, Brayne C, et al. Global prevalence of dementia: a Delphi consensus study. *Lancet*. 2005;**366**.

109. Leys D, Pasquier F, Parnetti L. Epidemiology of vascular dementia. *Haemostasis*. 1998;**28**:134–150.

110. Rizzi L, Rosset I, Roriz-Cruz M. Global epidemiology of dementia: Alzheimer's and vascular types. *BioMed Res Int*. 2014;1-8.

111. Lobo A, Launer LJ, Fratiglioni L, et al. Prevalence of dementia and major subtypes in Europe: a collaborative study of population-based cohorts. Neurologic Diseases in the Elderly Research Group. *Neurology*. 1999;**54**:S4–S9.

112. Ikeda M, Hokoishi K, Maki N, et al. Increased prevalence of vascular dementia in Japan: a community-based epidemiological study. *Neurology*. 2001;**57**:839–844.

113. Zhang Y, Xu Y, Nie H, et al. Prevalence of dementia and major dementia subtypes in the Chinese populations: a meta-analysis of dementia prevalence surveys, 1980–2010. *J Clin Neurosci: Off J Neurosurg Soc Australas*. 2012;**19**:1333–1337.

114. Pendlebury ST, Rothwell PM. Prevalence, incidence, and factors associated with pre-stroke and post-stroke dementia: a systematic review and meta-analysis. *Lancet Neurol*. 2009;**8**:1006–1018.

115. Levine DA, Galecki AT, Langa KM, et al. Trajectory of cognitive decline after incident stroke. *JAMA*. 2015;**314**:41–51.

116. Savva GM, Stephan BCM, Alzheimer's Society Vascular Dementia Systematic Review Group: epidemiological studies of the effect of stroke on incident dementia: a systematic review. *Stroke*. 2010;**41**:e41–e46.

117. Sposato LA, Kapral MK, Fang J, et al. Declining incidence of stroke and dementia: coincidence or prevention opportunity? *JAMA Neurol*. 2015;**72**:1529–1531.

118. Hachinski V, Sposato LA. Dementia: from muddled diagnoses to treatable mechanisms. *Brain: J Neurol*. 2013;**136**:2652–2654.

119. Gorelick PB, Scuteri A, Black SE, et al., American Heart Association Stroke Council, Council on Epidemiology and Prevention, Council on Cardiovascular Nursing, Council on Cardiovascular Radiology and Intervention, and Council on Cardiovascular Surgery and Anesthesia: Vascular contributions to cognitive impairment and dementia: a statement for healthcare professionals from the American Heart Association/American Stroke Association. *Stroke*. 2011;**42**:2672–2713.

120. Solomon A, Mangialasche F, Richard E, et al. Advances in the prevention of Alzheimer's disease and dementia. *J Intern Med*. 2014;**275**:229–250.

121. Román GC. Stroke, cognitive decline and vascular dementia: the silent epidemic of the 21st century. *Neuroepidemiology*. 2002;**22** (3):161–164.

122. Launer LJ, Petrovitch H, Ross GW, Markesbery W, White LR. AD brain pathology: vascular origins? Results from the HAAS autopsy study. *Neurobiol Aging*. 2008;**29**:1587–1590.

123. Iturria-Medina Y, Sotero RC, Toussaint PJ, Evans AC, Alzheimer's Disease Neuroimaging Initiative: Epidemic spreading model to characterize misfolded proteins propagation in aging and associated neurodegenerative

disorders. *PLoS Comput Biol.* 2014;**10**(11): e1003956.

124. Li L, Zhang X, Yang D, Luo G, Chen S, Le W. Hypoxia increases Abeta generation by altering beta- and gamma-cleavage of APP. *Neurobiol Aging.* 2009; **30**:1091–1098.

125. Bell RD, Zlokovic BV. Neurovascular mechanisms and blood-brain barrier disorder in Alzheimer's disease. *Acta Neuropathol.* 2009;**118**:103–113.

126. Iadecola C. Cerebrovascular effects of amyloid-beta peptides: mechanisms and implications for Alzheimer's dementia. *Cell Mol Neurobiol.* 2003;**23**:681–689.

Diagnosis of Potentially Preventable Dementias

José G. Merino and Clinton B. Wright

Introduction

The traditional diagnostic and therapeutic approach to patients with cognitive impairment and dementia has been to classify them into one of two broad groups: neurodegenerative conditions or vascular dementia. A few patients have been considered to have "reversible" dementias due to treatable conditions such as vitamin deficiencies, thyroid disease, subdural hematoma, normal pressure hydrocephalus, depression and medication side effects.[1] But, as detailed in other chapters in this book, the brains of most elderly people harbor both pathological hallmarks of neurodegenerative disorders (neurofibrillary tangles, amyloid plaques, diffuse Lewy bodies) and vascular changes, and these pathologies have synergistic effects.[2–4] In addition, vascular factors contribute to cognitive decline in patients traditionally considered to have Alzheimer disease. As a result, vascular cognitive impairment (VCI) may be the most common cause of preventable dementia.

VCI is a complex nosological concept that refers to "a heterogeneous group of conditions in which vascular factors are associated with or cause cognitive deficits."[5] This broad concept includes cognitive impairment of any severity (from the brain-at-risk stage to severe dementia) and is associated with, or caused by, any vascular pathology including "strokes, large and small,"[6] "silent" brain infarcts, microscopic infarcts, white matter pathology, cerebral microbleeds, chronic hypoperfusion, global ischemia, and mixed primary neurodegenerative and cerebrovascular pathologies.[7] The concept may also be extended to patients with cognitive impairment of a non-vascular etiology and significant vascular risk factors that place them at risk of such damage.

Our understanding of the interaction of vascular and neurodegenerative processes in the brain is evolving, and definite criteria to diagnose VCI have not yet been established.[8–10] But using VCI as a model to guide their diagnostic approach, clinicians may identify vascular factors that, if modified, can prevent, delay, or even reverse cognitive impairment. In this chapter, we describe an approach to patients with cognitive impairment that is based on The National Institute of Neurological Disorders and Stroke and the Canadian Stroke Network (NINDS-CSN) Harmonization Standards. This approach is helpful for clinicians when assessing patients with cognitive impairment and may help identify those patients in whom timely intervention may halt or reverse the cognitive decline.[9]

Clinical Evaluation

When faced with a patient with cognitive symptoms (or concerns) it is important to exclude conditions that are susceptible to therapeutic interventions, including cardiovascular and cerebrovascular disease (see Table 2.1). The NINDS-CSN harmonization standards identify

Table 2.1 DEMENTIA table to identify reversible dementias

Reversible, preventable and treatable subtypes of DEMENTIA	
D	Drugs: Polypharmacy, anticholinergics
E	Eye and ear deficits
M	Metabolic disorders
E	Emotion: Depression Endocrine: Hypothyroidism
N	Nutrition: Vitamin B12 deficiency Normal Pressure Hydrocephalus
T	Toxic Trauma Tumor
I	Ischemia / intracerebral hemorrhage Infection: HIV, neurosyphilis
A	Alcohol

Source: Tripathi M, Vibha D. Reversible dementia. Indian Journal of Psychiatry. 2009;51(Suppl. 1):S52–S55.

the most relevant demographic, anamnestic, clinical, neuropsychological, and imaging elements that may help identify patients with suspected VCI and this will be the focus of this chapter.

History of the Present Illness

The clinical history of the condition provides clues to establish the diagnosis of VCI and identify possible etiologic factors. The evaluation of the patient with cognitive impairment must include elucidation of the symptoms (cognitive and vascular), their duration and severity, and an assessment of the degree of insight into problems detected by others. Interviewing an informant who knows the subject well is recommended because the patients themselves often lack insight into their condition, especially when it involves memory. In addition, some patients may deny a history of discrete stroke or VCI, but detailed questioning about signs and symptoms suggestive of these conditions may yield important information about unrecognized cerebrovascular disease. Important anamnestic factors recommended by the NINDS CSN Harmonization Standards include demographics, health history, and family history.

The nature and severity of the symptoms, and the cognitive functions affected, depend on the type, extent, and location of the cerebrovascular changes and, if present, the neurodegenerative pathology. Patients with single cortical infarcts may have deficits in specific higher brain functions (language, praxis, attention) while those with more extensive subcortical pathology (or with strategically placed single infarcts) that disrupt distributed brain networks may have difficulties with information processing, planning, learning, and memory retrieval. The timing of onset of symptoms and the rate of progression, as well as recognition of any precipitating events (including surgery) yield clues about the etiology of the cognitive impairment. In some patients, particularly those with cortical or strategically placed infarcts, the disease is characterized by stepwise deterioration associated with clinical strokes. This is the classical multi-infarct dementia phenotype.[11] But most patients will have a more gradual onset and progression. This pattern is seen most often, but not exclusively, in patients with multiple small vessel infarcts that involve the basal ganglia and the thalamus or those with extensive changes of the white matter and those with mixed pathologies.[8] When progression is gradual, patients and families may not seek medical attention until the cognitive impairment is severe because they adapt to these changes and may consider them a part of normal aging. Since vascular damage acts synergistically with Alzheimer pathology, a slow progressive course does not eliminate the opportunity to treat vascular disease.

Patients with mild VCI often complain of difficulties in "executive function." They take longer to plan or complete tasks and have trouble multitasking. Some find that they have to work longer hours to complete their job duties, or that they have difficulty keeping up with household activities such as balancing their bank account or planning their day. In the early stages, they may use compensatory strategies (such as making lists), but later they have to rely on caregivers to help them make decisions. Patients who were fastidious about their appearance may become slovenly and others may undergo personality changes. The patient's spouse or friends may notice that they repeat themselves, have word-finding difficulties, make paraphasic errors, or have trouble with comprehension. Some patients with VCI have short-term memory problems; others may get lost in familiar places. When these symptoms appear early in the course of the disease, neurodegenerative conditions must be considered.[12] Over time, as these deficits become more pronounced, they interfere with social and professional activities and, in the later stages, once dementia develops, patients need help performing ADLs and require constant supervision. Eventually they become completely dependent on others.

Patients with cognitive impairment after a clinical stroke represent a specific subgroup within VCI. Three months after a stroke, up to one-third of patients meet criteria for vascular dementia.[13] An even higher proportion of patients may have milder cognitive impairment, and in some the deficits are temporary. Almost half of the patients with lacunar stroke enrolled in the Secondary Prevention of Small Subcortical Strokes trial had some degree of cognitive impairment at the time of enrollment, even if they did not have residual sensory or motor symptoms from the stroke.[14] In addition, approximately 10 percent to 15 percent of patients with post-stroke dementia may have pre-existing cognitive impairment and these patients may have a higher risk of having post-stroke dementia.[13]

The Ischemic Score (for further information refer to Hachinski et al. Arch of Neuro. 1975;32:632-637 and for scoring system get in touch with vladimir.hachinski@lhsc.on.ca) was developed to differentiate patients with multi-infarct dementia from those with Alzheimer disease and takes into account clinical factors such as the course of the cognitive impairment, the presence of risk factors, and the findings on the neurological examination;[15] it has 90 percent sensitivity and specificity to differentiate multi-infarct dementia and Alzheimer disease, but it is much less useful for differentiating mixed dementia.[16]

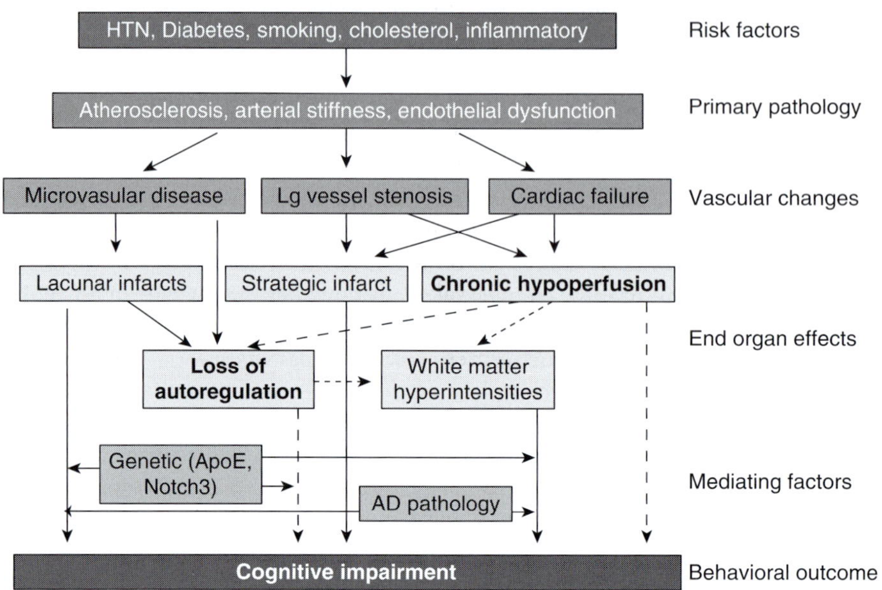

Figure 2.1 Model for the pathophysiology of cognitive impairment. Dotted lines indicate potentially reversible hemodynamic pathways.

Past Medical History

When evaluating a patient with suspected VCI, it is important to identify the presence of vascular risk factors and the age at which they became manifest, because numerous epidemiological studies have found an association between a history of metabolic syndrome, smoking, obesity, physical inactivity, poor diet, less or more than moderate alcohol consumption, hypertension, hyperlipidemia, diabetes mellitus, and insulin resistance at midlife and cognitive impairment, including VCI and Alzheimer disease, in later decades.[7,17] These risk factors increase the risk of clinical stroke, subclinical cerebrovascular disease, and dementia (Figure 2.1).[7,18,19] Interventions to address these risk factors may prevent recurrent stroke. While treatment of some of these risk factors can lower the risk of clinical outcomes such as stroke, myocardial infarction, and death, a benefit on VCI has not been shown, perhaps because studies have used tests insensitive to the most relevant cognitive domains. Newer trials, such as the Systolic Pressure Intervention Trial (SPRINT), have been designed to detect dementia and cognitive changes using sensitive measures and informant interviews.

Another equally important consideration is the prescription drugs and health supplements that a patient is taking. Medications indicated for psychiatric and neurologic problems are often obvious potential offenders, but their frequent misuse even by experienced physicians is noteworthy. Benzodiazepines, for example, are often prescribed for everything from chronic anxiety to sleep problems.[20] Given their amnestic properties, their tendency to exacerbate sleep disorders (which can also contribute to cognitive problems), and their addictive properties, the indication for drugs in this class should be carefully considered. For example, short acting benzodiazepines such as alprazolam should not be used for insomnia, or given multiple times per day to control generalized anxiety. Other classes of drugs whose indication should be questioned are opiates (for pain control) and antiepileptic drugs (to control symptoms such as mood lability). But, commonly prescribed drugs meant to treat other medical conditions can also be problematic in those at risk of cognitive impairment. Several studies have shown the potentially negative effects of drugs with anticholinergic properties that penetrate the CNS with strong anticholinergics showing an increased risk of dementia.[21] Many of these drugs are quite common, including those for cardiac disease and hypertension (e.g., many beta adrenergic receptor blockers), allergies, and genitourinary problems. Statin use has become very prevalent in developed countries and a number of studies have raised questions about their negative cognitive effects (although some evidence suggests they may be beneficial as a class, large randomized clinical trials have been negative).

Family History

Details of the family history are important in assessing the risk of both complex genetic diseases and those that follow classical Mendelian patterns. For example, a family history of Alzheimer disease in a first-degree relative confers increased risk of dementia and makes it more likely that the disease may be playing a role in VCI. Other disorders that are relevant to VCI include genetic forms of cerebral small vessel disease such as Cerebral Autosomal-Dominant Arteriopathy with Subcortical Infarcts and Leukoencephalopathy (CADASIL), cerebral autosomal recessive arteriopathy with subcortical infarcts and leukoencephalopathy (CARASIL), autosomal dominant retinal vasculopathy with cerebral leukodystrophy, *COL4A1* cerebral small vessel disease, and Fabry disease.[22] While not preventable at this time, testing should be considered in adults below age 50 with cognitive decline along with other characteristic features that are disease-specific. In CADASIL, brain imaging with MRI often shows white matter lesions in the temporal poles, whereas in CARASIL hyperintensities are more often periventricular with sparing of U-fibers.[22] Genetic testing for mutations in the *NOTCH3* gene in CADASIL and the *HTRA1* gene in CARASIL should be considered in appropriate cases, and a skin biopsy should be considered in CADASIL (In CARASIL skin lesions are less ubiquitous). Fabry disease is caused by deficient or absent lysosomal α-galactosidase A activity and has protean manifestations. Acroparesthesias are quite characteristic and often seen in childhood, along with abdominal pain, angiokeratomas, and dyshydrosis. Later, impaired renal function and heart disease complicate the picture, adding cardioembolic stroke to the list of brain insults a Fabry patient may suffer in addition to the cerebral small vessel disease itself. Enzyme replacement therapy has revolutionized treatment of this disease.[22]

Physical Examination

The physical examination can provide objective evidence of cardiac, vascular, and cerebrovascular disease and other conditions associated with VCI and may help differentiate patients with VCI from those with other causes of cognitive impairment. The evaluation of patients with suspected VCI must include a detailed examination of the cardiovascular system looking for evidence of heart failure, rhythm abnormalities, structural heart abnormalities, and carotid or peripheral vascular disease because cerebral hypoperfusion due to carotid artery occlusion, congestive heart failure, and microvascular disease may lead to cognitive impairment that in some instances may be reversible.[23,24] Any abnormality detected on the examination will require confirmation with ancillary studies including carotid imaging, electrocardiography, long-term cardiac rhythm monitoring and echocardiography.

Neurological Examination

The neurological examination provides important etiologic clues in patients with cognitive decline. Patients with large artery strokes have evidence of focal brain lesions on examination: hemiparesis with increased muscular tone, hemisensory loss, visual field and other cranial nerve deficits, unilateral incoordination, asymmetric and/or brisk reflexes, an extensor plantar response (Babinski sign) or unsteadiness of gait. When the cerebrovascular pathology affects subcortical structures including the basal ganglia, thalamus, and white matter tracts, in addition to hemiparesis and sensory changes, patients may have prominent early gait changes (marche à petits pas or a magnetic, apraxic or Parkinsonian gait), frequent falls, urinary frequency or incontinence, and pseudobulbar palsy (upper motor neuron weakness of the face, tongue and pharynx, spastic dysarthria, dysphagia, and emotional incontinence). These features of subcortical disease are rare in patients with Alzheimer disease until later stages of the disease.

Mental Status Examination

The location of cerebrovascular lesions may explain the presenting neurocognitive syndrome in patients with VCI. Medial frontal infarcts may produce executive dysfunction, abulia, apathy, and, when lesions are bilateral, akinetic mutism. Medial temporal lesions may cause amnesia. Infarcts of the left lateral frontal or parietal lobes may cause aphasia, agnosia, and apraxia while lesions in the corresponding areas of the right hemisphere lead to hemineglect, anosognosia, asomatognosia, confusion, agitation, and visuospatial and constructional difficulties.[25] Strategically placed subcortical infarcts may mimic cortical lesions because they interrupt frontal-subcortical neural networks. Extensive subcortical disease is characterized by abulia, apathy and emotional incontinence, and a more diffuse process affecting several domains, particularly but not exclusively those related to executive function.[26] Patients with significant co-existing Alzheimer-type pathology may have memory loss and a clinical picture consistent with Alzheimer disease. Because subcortical lesions also disrupt thalamocortical, striatocapsular, and prefrontal-basal ganglia pathways, patients with VCI often have behavioral and mood disorders. Depression and apathy are particularly common in patients with VaD while hallucinations and delusions are in AD.[27] But these features are not specific to a vascular etiology.[12] In addition, a third of stroke patients may have mood changes a few months after a stroke, and depression may mimic VCI.

Many of these signs and symptoms can be elicited through a detailed clinical mental status examination, and readers are referred to standard neurology textbooks for reference. Standardized scales and tests may also aid in the bedside evaluation of these patients and may highlight subtle cognitive changes and help track disease progression. It is important to use scales and tools that are sensitive to a variety of cognitive domains, particularly executive function. The Montreal Cognitive Assessment (MoCA) is a good screening instrument for

VCI that is free and available online (www.mocatest.org).[28] It can be completed in 10 minutes and evaluates 8 cognitive domains: visuospatial/executive functions, naming, memory, attention, language, abstraction, and orientation. It is particularly well suited for patients with mild VCI because five of the eight items focus on executive function.[29] It is also helpful to assess cognition in patients after stroke.[30] The NINDS-CSN Harmonization Criteria recommend the use of some tests in the MoCA as a quick screening tool that takes less than five minutes to administer: a six-word memory task (registration, recall, recognition), six-item orientation, and one-letter phonemic fluency.[9] The Frontal Assessment Battery (FAB) and the VADASCog-Vascular dementia assessment scale are sensitive to vascular damage and can identify frontal dysexecutive syndromes.[31,32] While the most frequently used test in routine practice is the Folstein Mini-Mental State Examination (MMSE), it is important to remember that it was developed to identify patients with Alzheimer disease, and it is not sensitive for subtle executive dysfunction.[33,34] It also has a ceiling effect and patients with MCI may score in the normal range (≥ 25). Copyright protection for this test is now enforced, and it must be purchased from the publisher (www .parinc.com).

Neuropsychological Evaluation

A detailed neuropsychological evaluation is necessary to identify the specific cognitive domains affected and the severity of the impairment. Repeat examinations several months or years apart can be used to track the course of disease and evaluate the impact of any interventions. The pattern of impaired cognitive domains may help differentiate VCI from neurodegenerative conditions (including Alzheimer disease, dementia with Lewy bodies, and fronto-temporal dementia) and identify patients with depression and other mood disorders. A brief psychiatric inventory or depression screen, such as the Centers for Epidemiologic Study of Depression (CES-D) or the Geriatric Depression Scale (GDS) can be useful to identify significant depressive symptomatology.

Neuropsychological batteries must be comprehensive but include several tests of executive function because this cognitive domain is often affected in patients with VCI. The NINDS-CSN Harmonization Criteria recommend specific protocols that can be used in different settings: an extensive protocol (that takes about one hour to administer) to fully evaluate patients with VCI, a shorter protocol (~30 minutes) that may be used for clinical screening, and the very brief protocol described above that can be applied at the bedside or in the office.[9] The longer batteries must be administered by a neuropsychologist. Standardized tools for detecting neuropsychiatric abnormalities are also available. While a discussion of these test batteries is beyond the scope of this chapter, specific batteries are listed in Table 2.2 for reference.

Neuroimaging

Neuroimaging is required to support a diagnosis of VCI and to exclude other conditions that can lead to cognitive impairment including tumors, infections, traumatic subdural hemorrhage, and normal pressure hydrocephalus. But VCI is a heterogeneous condition without pathognomonic imaging findings and neuroimaging is therefore descriptive rather than diagnostic. CT scanners are widely available and can show evidence of larger subacute and chronic infarcts and extensive white matter changes but may not be sensitive to mild

Table 2.2 NINDS-CSN harmonization criteria neuropsych evaluation list

Sixty-Minute Neuropsychological Protocol
Executive/Activation
Animal Naming (semantic fluency)
Controlled Oral Word Association Test
WAIS-III Digit Symbol-Coding
Trailmaking Test
List Learning Test Strategies
Future Use: Simple and Choice Reaction Time
Language/Lexical Retrieval
Boston Naming Test 2nd Edition, Short Form
Visuospatial
Rey-Osterrieth Complex Figure Copy
Supplemental: Complex Figure Memory
Memory
Hopkins Verbal Learning Test-Revised
Alternate: California Verbal Learning Test–2
Supplemental: Boston Naming Test Recognition
Supplemental: Digit Symbol- Coding Incidental Learning
Neuropsychiatric/Depressive Symptoms
Neuropsychiatric Inventory - Questionnaire Version (NPI-Q)
Center for Epidemiological Studies-Depression Scale
Other
Informant Questionnaire for Cognitive Decline in the Elderly
MMSE
Thirty Minute Test Protocol
Semantic Fluency (Animal Naming)
Phonemic Fluency (Controlled Oral Word Association Test)
Digit Symbol-Coding from the Wechsler Adult Intelligence Scale, Third Edition
Hopkins Verbal Learning Test
Center for Epidemiologic Studies-Depression Scale

Table 2.2 (cont.)

Neuropsychiatric Inventory, Questionnaire Version (NPI-Q)
Supplemental: MMSE, Trail Making Test
Five Minute Protocol
Montreal Cognitive Assessment MoCA subtests
5-Word Memory Task (registration, recall, recognition)
6-Item Orientation
1-Letter Phonemic Fluency

Supplemental: Remainder of the MoCA, Semantic Fluency (Animal Naming), Trail Making Test, MMSE (to be administered at least 1 hour before or after the above tests).
Source: Hachinski V, Iadecola C, Petersen RC, et al. National Institute of Neurological Disorders and Stroke-Canadian Stroke Network vascular cognitive impairment harmonization standards. Stroke. 2006;37(9): 2220–2241.

disease. The findings are difficult to quantify, and they expose the patient to significant radiation. Magnetic resonance imaging (MRI) is a better imaging tool in this setting. Different MRI sequences provide important information. T1-weighted, T2-weighted, and fluid inversion recovery (FLAIR) sequences provide information about the anatomy and the presence of atrophy and other chronic pathologies; diffusion-weighted imaging (DWI) can visualize areas of acute infarction; T2*-weighted gradient-echo recalled (GRE) scans can

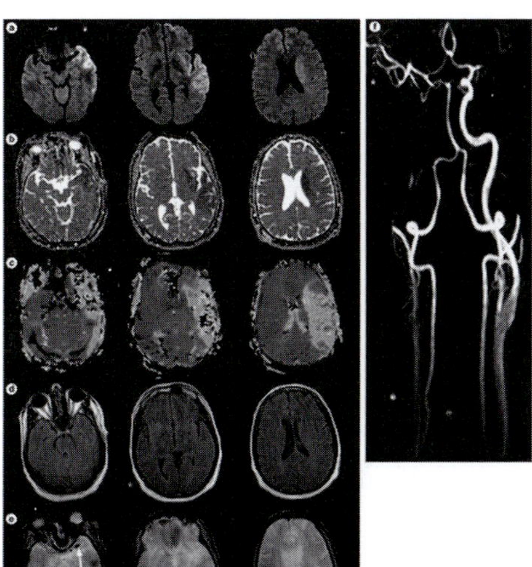

Figure 2.2 Acute MRI scan.[58]
Source: Merino JG, Warach S. Imaging of acute stroke. *Nature reviews Neurology* 2010;6(10):560–571.

identify acute and chronic micro- and macro-bleeds; and perfusion-weighted images (PWI) identify abnormalities in brain perfusion. Magnetic resonance angiography allows visualization of the patency of intra- and extra-cranial vessels. (see Figure 2.2). Below we address some of the more significant pathologic changes that are seen in patients with VCI. It is important to remember that no single neuroimaging abnormality by itself is sufficient or required to diagnose VCI. Not all vascular lesions seen on neuroimaging are sufficient to cause VCI, and not all vascular lesions that may contribute to VCI are readily seen on neuroimaging because they can be below the resolution of specific scans.[35]

Brain infarction is the most important cerebrovascular pathology that contributes to cognitive impairment. As discussed above, up to a third of patients who have a stroke have evidence of cognitive impairment three months after the stroke. There is no clear volume threshold of damage that is both necessary and sufficient to diagnose VCI, but the risk of cognitive impairment increases when larger or multiple infarcts are present. While a single large infarct may lead to cognitive impairment, smaller infarcts in the subcortical white matter or gray nuclei also lead to cognitive impairment if they are multiple or, if single, they disrupt key cortical-subcortical circuits.[12] Such strategic locations include the left angular gyrus, inferomesial temporal and mesial frontal lobes, anterior and dorsomedial thalamus, left capsular genu, and caudate nucleus.[36] Lacunar infarcts contribute to cognitive impairment in patients with VCI and mixed pathology. On CT, they are hypodense subcortical lesions. On T1- or T2-weighted MRI, they may appear as a small round or ovoid hypointense lesions (3–15 mm), but on FLAIR they may have a hyperintense rim because of perilesional gliosis or may appear hyperintense if the central cavity fluid is not suppressed by FLAIR. Lacunes must be differentiated from enlarged Virchow-Robbins spaces, the CSF-filled spaces that surround vessels as they enter the brain parenchyma. While they are also hypointense on T1- and T2-weighted sequences, when seen on adjacent slices they may have an elongated shape and are most often seen in the basal ganglia (Figure 2.3).[37] Infraputaminal lacunes can be mistaken for infarcts but have been shown in pathological studies to be enlarged perivascular spaces (Figure 2.4).[38]

Some patients without a history of clinical stroke have infarcts on brain imaging. The prevalence of these "silent" infarcts increases with age. In the Framingham cohort, for example, they were present in ~10 percent of those in their 5th to 7th decade, 17 percent in those in the 8th decade, and 30 percent of those older than 80.[39] Careful anamnesis and examination may reveal the presence of subtle symptoms and signs of a stroke, and patients with these lesions have a high risk of developing dementia and rapid cognitive decline.[40] These "silent" infarcts, particularly when accompanied by white matter changes, may be a surrogate marker that can be used to identify patients at risk for VCI.[8]

Changes in the white matter are highly prevalent dementia in the elderly. They appear as hypodense areas on CT. On MRI, they are hypointense on T1-weighted sequences and hyperintense on T2-weighted scans. Because they are often seen along the periventricular border, they are best visualized with FLAIR, a T2-weighted sequence that suppresses CSF signal and makes the ventricles appear dark. These changes may be focal or multifocal and may involve most of the white matter. The prevalence of these changes increases with age and the presence of midlife risk factors, but they are also seen in

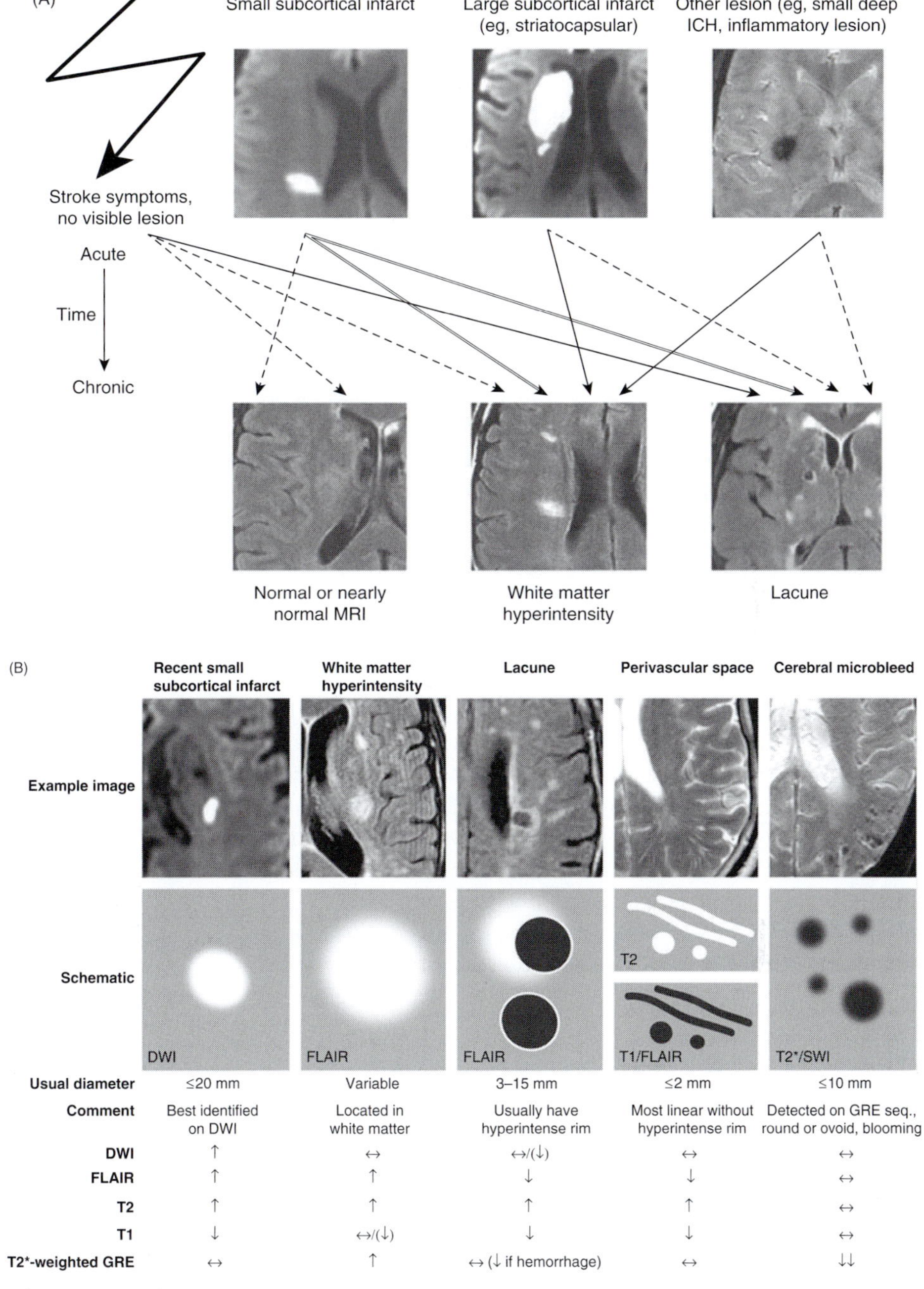

Figure 2.3 Findings on MRI.
A. Variable fates of lesions related to small vessel disease and the convergence of acute lesions with different causes but similar late appearances on MRI
Arrows indicate possible late fates of acute MRI findings. Double lines indicate common fates of recent small subcortical infarcts, dashed lines indicate less common fates, and solid lines indicate least common late fates. ICH = intracranial hemorrhage.
B. MRI findings for lesions related to small vessel disease.
Shows examples (upper) and schematic representation (middle) of MRI features for changes related to small vessel disease, with a summary of imaging characteristics (lower) for individual lesions. DWI = diffusion-weighted imaging. FLAIR = fluid-attenuated inversion recovery. SWI = susceptibility-weighted imaging. GRE = gradient-recalled echo.
Reproduced with the kind permission of Elsevier from: Wardlaw JM, Smith EE, Biessels GJ, et al. Neuroimaging standards for research into small vessel disease and its contribution to ageing and neurodegeneration. *The Lancet Neurology* 2013;12(8):822–838.

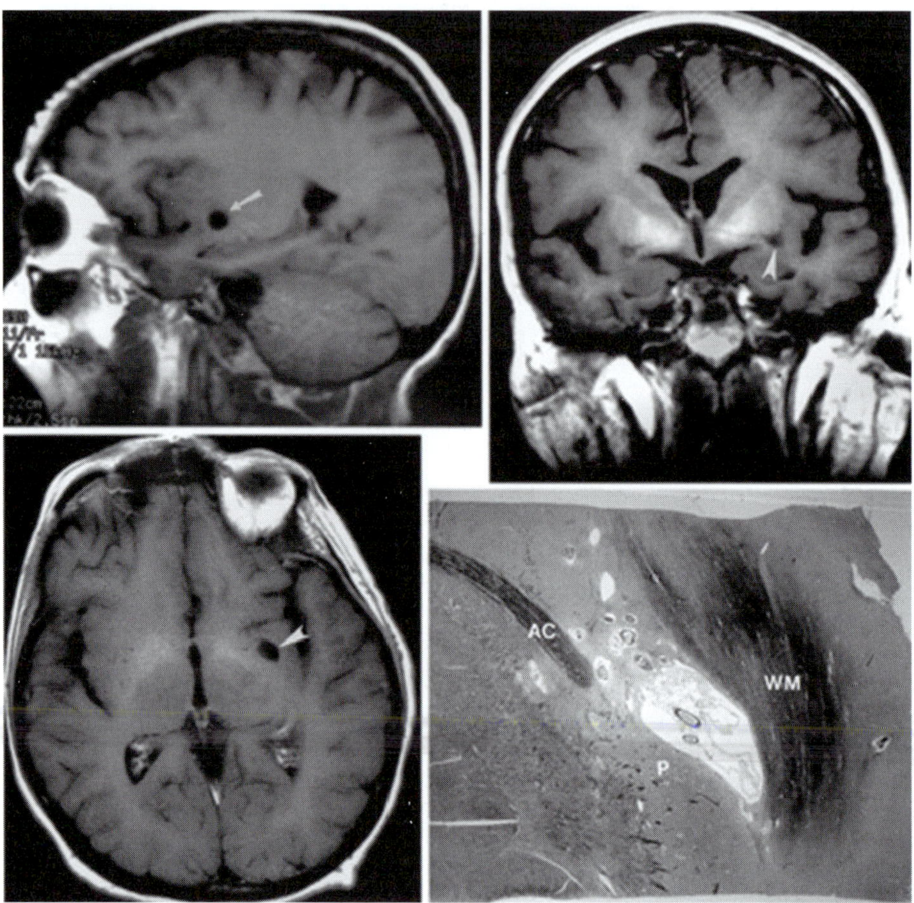

Figure 2.4 Infraputaminal lacunes are enlarged perivascular spaces but are often mistaken for lacunar infarcts on brain imaging. Reproduced with permission from Pullicino PM, Miller LL, Alexandrov AV, et al. Infraputaminal "Lacunes": clinical and pathological correlations. *Stroke.* 1995;26(9):1598–1602.

patients with multiple sclerosis, migraine, brain tumors, and a history of brain irradiation, as well as patients with mild vascular cognitive impairment, VCI, Alzheimer disease, dementia with Lewy bodies, and fronto-temporal dementias. While several scales have been developed for use in research studies, in routine clinical practice their extent is not often quantified. Because they are so prevalent, particularly in the elderly, it is difficult to determine their impact on an individual patient but epidemiologic studies show that when extensive, they are associated with a doubling of the risk of dementia.[12,41] The cause for these changes in many patients is assumed to be demyelination with axonal loss, gliosis and disruption of the blood-brain barrier due to chronic ischemia caused by arteriolosclerosis, lipohyalinosis, and fibrinoid necrosis of penetrating vessels.[37,42] These white matter changes are often associated with thinning of the cortex and disruption of white matter tracts.[42]

Intracranial hemorrhage may be associated with cognitive impairment. Up to two-thirds of survivors of a subarachnoid hemorrhage have residual cognitive impairment. Intraparenchymal hemorrhage may have an effect similar to that of ischemic stroke on the subsequent development of VCI. Several hereditary conditions associated with cerebral amyloid angiopathy (CAA) and other genetic conditions can present as multiple hemorrhages, and carry an increased risk of VCI. In addition, many patients harbor one or more cerebral microbleeds (CMB): small (up to 10 mm) areas of signal void associated with blooming artifact on T2*-weighted MRI sequences such as GRE.[43] These lesions are not well seen on CT. In pathological studies, these lesions are associated with hemosiderin deposits suggestive of small chronic hemorrhages. They can be seen in patients with Alzheimer disease (often in association with CAA), VCI, and in those with normal cognition. Patients with hypertension often have one or more CMBs in the deep nuclei, the basal ganglia, and the thalamus. In patients with CAA, these CMBs tend to be located in the cortex, at the junction of the gray and white matter, predominately in posterior areas of the brain. Evidence of superficial siderosis on T2* GRE is also common in those with CAA.

Atrophy of mesial temporal lobes is typically seen in AD but also in patients with VCI. Hippocampal atrophy may result from a mixture of ischemic and degenerative pathologies. The cause of the atrophy is not known, but it may be related to abnormalities in the subjacent white matter.[42,44] There may be a synergistic interaction between white matter changes, atrophy, and cognition.[45] Most clinical radiology reports do not include details about hippocampal atrophy (but often radiologists will comment on global atrophy).

Functional imaging studies can help differentiate patients with VCI and Alzheimer disease and also help evaluate the independent and combined effects of vascular and AD brain injury during aging.[8] PET can be used to image glucose metabolic rates using 18F Fluorodeoxyglucose. Patients with Alzheimer disease have decreased bilateral temporal and parietal uptake while patients with VCI have patchy abnormalities. A 11C-labelled PET tracer, the Pittsburgh Compound B (or PiB) can detect the fibrillary form of amyloid plaques and can help detect patients with Alzheimer-type pathology.[46] This tracer also binds vascular amyloid and can identify patients with CAA. These imaging modalities are predominately used for research at this time.

Laboratory Evaluation

Metabolic, nutritional, and endocrine abnormalities may contribute to cognitive impairment. The initial evaluation of patients with cognitive complaints must include a comprehensive metabolic panel (electrolytes and liver and renal function tests), thyroid function tests (at minimum, TSH), and vitamin B12 and homocysteine levels. Any identified abnormalities may require further evaluation. Depending on the clinical features, additional tests may be required including an inflammatory screen (ANA, ESR, CRP), tests for infectious agents (HIV, Lyme), a paraneoplastic antibody screen, Whipples PCR and measurement of ceruloplasmin, serum and urinary copper, and a urinary heavy metal screen. Analysis of CSF may be useful in some patients and in addition to cell count and chemistry, may include tests for treponemal antibodies, cryptococcal antigen, stains and cultures for bacterial and fungal agents, stains for acid-fast bacilli, cytology, viral PCR and cultures, Lyme antibodies, and 14-3-3 proteins. In patients suspected of a genetic form of vascular problems, testing for the presence of genetic variants may be warranted.[8]

Several biomarkers of Alzheimer disease pathology (amyloid detected on PET, amyloid-tau biomarkers in CSF and genetic studies) can help differentiate patients with Alzheimer disease from those with VCI and mixed dementia.[8] Work is ongoing to identify additional serum and CSF biomarkers that may help in the early diagnosis and monitoring of progression in patients with VCI. Relevant associations have been found for serum biomarkers related to inflammation, endothelial dysfunction with blood-brain barrier abnormalities and breakdown of the neurovascular unit, hemostasis, and components of the renin-angiotensin-aldosterone system.[47-49] We expect that in the future a combination of these tests may be used to identify specific subgroups of VCI patients. At present, however, these tests are not used routinely in the clinical setting.

Diagnosis of VCI

The diagnosis of VCI relies on a combination of clinical, neuropsychological, and radiological features, but because there are no pathognomonic characteristics of VCI – no single characteristic, even neuropathological findings, is diagnostic in any individual case – the development of diagnostic criteria has been challenging.[8,9] One of the key limiting factors has been the difficulty in establishing the amount of vascular damage both necessary and sufficient to cause cognitive impairment. In the 1990s, several groups developed criteria for vascular dementia to be used in research studies.[50-54] These criteria have several limitations. They only identify patients in the later stages of disease and, because they are based on the Alzheimer paradigm, identify only patients with prominent memory impairment. Because they require a clinical or radiological temporal association with stroke, they primarily identify patients with post-stroke dementia. More recent diagnostic models recognize the heterogeneity of the VCI concept and take a less rigid approach to diagnosis, allowing for a broader range of severity and impairment of any cognitive domain (e.g., executive function, attention, psychomotor speed). The Diagnostic and Statistical Manual, 5th Edition (DSM-5), classifies patients with cognitive impairment into two groups defined by severity: major (fulfilling the criteria for dementia) and mild neurocognitive syndrome. Any cognitive domain may be affected, and cerebrovascular disease is accepted as a potential cause of these syndromes.[55] A Statement for Healthcare Professionals from the American Heart Association / American Stroke Association defines VCI as "a syndrome with evidence of clinical stroke or subclinical vascular brain injury and cognitive impairment affecting at least one cognitive domain." The authors of this statement propose a practical approach and criteria to classify patients with suspected VCI.[8] They differentiate vascular dementia (VaD; a decline in cognitive function from a prior baseline and a deficit in performance in two or more cognitive domains that impair the patient's ability to perform activities of daily living [ADL]) from vascular mild cognitive impairment (VaMCI; where one or more cognitive domains may be affected and patients are able to perform ADLs). They propose two categories for each diagnosis, probable or possible, depending on the certainty of the relationship between the vascular disease and onset of cognitive deficits (timing, severity, or cognitive pattern). These may be more suitable for research. Other groups have proposed diagnostic subtypes of VCI such as multi-infarct dementia and dementia from subcortical ischemic small vessel disease.[11,26] Ongoing initiatives aim to develop harmonization standards and define a set of data elements to be collected in future studies aimed at more fully defining VCI, understanding its etiology, and identifying targets for treatment. As our understanding grows, it is likely that the diagnostic criteria will be modified.[9]

Conclusion

Vascular cognitive impairment (VCI) is the most common cause of preventable dementia, and it is important for clinicians to recognize any vascular pathology and risk factors in patients who are being evaluated for cognitive complaints of any severity. An approach to patients based on the NINDS-CSN harmonization standards may help clinicians faced with these patients.

"Guideline-Based Approach to Vascular Cognitive Impairment

A history of vascular disease or poorly controlled risk factors may increase the likelihood of VCI. Based on the American Heart Association / American Stroke Association Statement, patients presenting with possible VCI/VaMCI and cognitive complaints should be evaluated with formal neurocognitive testing in cases where impairment is suspected. Once cognitive impairment has been determined, brain imaging must be present to qualify for VCI. For VaMCI, the criteria are similar but activities of daily living limitations must be at most mild, or explained by noncognitive deficits related to an underlying disease, including stroke (e.g., motor or sensory deficits).

a) A documented history of stroke or neuroimaging evidence of vascular damage is required by American Heart Association / American Stroke Association criteria. A screening test such as the Montreal Cognitive Assessment (MoCA) may be used to decide if formal testing should be done. If cognitive impairment is suspected, formal neurocognitive testing should be done. Brain imaging should be used to substantiate vascular damage, preferably brain MRI on a closed magnet with field strength of at least 1.5 Tesla. However, in some cases computed tomography of the head may be substituted when MR is contra-indicated or cannot be tolerated.

b) Activity of daily living assessments that evaluate the patient's ability to carry out instrumental (higher order) functions, such as managing finances, preparing meals, and shopping, should be determined by using a structured questionnaire and a reliable informant. Devices such as the Functional Activities Questionnaire (FAQ) or the Informant Questionnaire on Cognitive Decline in the Elderly (IQCODE) can help determine if there are major deficits in function. Such deficits in combination with considerable cognitive impairment help distinguish between VaMCI and VaD.

c) Evidence of Alzheimer disease biology includes positive amyloid imaging using positron emission tomography or spinal fluid biomarkers (amyloid/tau ratio and elevated phosphorylated tau)."

References

1. Kabasakalian A, Finney GR. Reversible dementias. *Int Rev Neurobiol.* 2009;**84**:283–302.

2. Snowdon DA, Greiner LH, Mortimer JA, et al. Brain infarction and the clinical expression of Alzheimer disease: The Nun Study. *JAMA* 1997;**277**(10):813–7

3. Neuropathology Group. Medical Research Council Cognitive Function and Aging Study Pathological correlates of late-onset dementia in a multicentre, community-based population in England and Wales. Neuropathology Group of the Medical Research Council Cognitive Function and Ageing Study (MRC CFAS). *Lancet* 2001;**357**(9251):169–175.

4. Toledo JB, Arnold SE, Raible K, et al. Contribution of cerebrovascular disease in autopsy confirmed neurodegenerative disease cases in the National Alzheimer's Coordinating Centre. *Brain.* 2013;**136**(Pt 9):2697–2706.

5. Bowler JB, Hachinski V. Vascular cognitive impairment: a new approach to vascular dementia. *Baillieres Clin Neurol* 1995;**4**:357–376.

6. Fisher CM. Dementia in cerebrovascular disease. In: Toole J, Siekert RJW, eds. *Cerebrovascular disease, The 6th Princeton Conference.* New York, NY: Grune & Stratton, 1968:232–241.

7. Gardener H, Wright CB, Rundek T, et al. Brain health and shared risk factors for dementia and stroke. *Nature Rev Neurol.* 2015;**11**(11):651–657.

8. Gorelick PB, Scuteri A, Black SE, et al. Vascular contributions to cognitive impairment and dementia: a statement for healthcare professionals from the American Heart Association/American Stroke Association. *Stroke.* 2011;**42**(9):2672–2713.

9. Hachinski V, Iadecola C, Petersen RC, et al. National Institute of Neurological Disorders and Stroke-Canadian Stroke Network vascular cognitive impairment harmonization standards. *Stroke.* 2006;**37**(9):2220–2241.

10. Raz L, Knoefel J, Bhaskar K. The neuropathology and cerebrovascular mechanisms of dementia. *J Cereb Blood Flow Metab.* 2016;**36**(1):172–186.

11. Hachinski VC, Lassen NA, Marshall J. Multi-infarct dementia: a cause of mental deterioration in the elderly. *Lancet.* 1974;**2**(7874):207–210.

12. Sachdev P, Kalaria R, O'Brien J, et al. Diagnostic criteria for vascular cognitive disorders: a VASCOG statement. *Alzheimer Dis Assoc Dis.* 2014;**28**(3):206–218.

13. Merino JG, Hachinski V. Stroke-related dementia. *Curr Atherosclerosis Reps.* 2002;**4**(4):285–290.

14. Jacova C, Pearce LA, Costello R, et al. Cognitive impairment in lacunar strokes: the SPS3 trial. *Ann Neurol.* 2012;**72**(3):351–362.

15. Hachinski VC, Iliff LD, Zilhka E, et al. Cerebral blood flow in dementia. *Arch Neurol.* 1975;**32**(9):632–637.

16. Moroney JT, Bagiella E, Desmond DW, et al. Meta-analysis of the Hachinski Ischemic Score in pathologically verified dementias. *Neurology.* 1997;**49**(4):1096–1105.

17. Luchsinger JA, Reitz C, Honig LS, et al. Aggregation of vascular risk factors and risk of incident Alzheimer disease. *Neurology.* 2005;**65**(4):545–551.

18. Rincon F, Wright CB. Vascular cognitive impairment. *Current Opin Neurol.* 2013;**26** (1):29–36.

19. Vieira JR, Elkind MS, Moon YP, et al. The metabolic syndrome and cognitive performance: the Northern Manhattan Study. *Neuroepidemiology.* 2011;**37**(3–4):153–159.

20. Airagnes G, Pelissolo A, Lavallee M, et al. Benzodiazepine misuse in the elderly: risk factors, consequences, and management. *Curr Psychiatry Reps.* 2016;**18**(10):89.

21. Gray SL, Anderson ML, Dublin S, et al. Cumulative use of strong anticholinergics and incident dementia: a prospective cohort study. *JAMA Intern Med.* 2015;**175** (3):401–407.

22. Federico A, Di Donato I, Bianchi S, et al. Hereditary cerebral small vessel diseases: a review. *J Neurol Sci.* 2012;**322** (1–2):25–30.

23. Marshall RS, Lazar RM. Pumps, aqueducts, and drought management: vascular physiology in vascular cognitive impairment. *Stroke.* 2011;**42**(1): 221–6.

24. Suemoto CK, Nitrini R, Grinberg LT, et al. Atherosclerosis and dementia: a cross-sectional study with pathological analysis of the carotid arteries. *Stroke.* 2011;**42**(12):3614–3615.

25. Funahashi S, Andreau JM. Prefrontal cortex and neural mechanisms of executive function. *J Physiol*, Paris, 2013;**107** (6):471–482.

26. Rosenberg GA, Wallin A, Wardlaw JM, et al. Consensus statement for diagnosis of subcortical small vessel disease. *J Cereb Blood Flow Metab.* 2016;**36**(1):6–25.

27. Lyketsos CG, Lopez O, Jones B, et al. Prevalence of neuropsychiatric symptoms in dementia and mild cognitive impairment: results from the Cardiovascular Health Study. *JAMA.* 2002;**288**(12):1475–1483.

28. Nasreddine ZS, Phillips NA, Bedirian V, et al. The Montreal Cognitive Assessment, MoCA: a brief screening tool for mild cognitive impairment. *J Am Geriatr Soc.* 2005;**53**(4):695–6p9.

29. Waldron-Perrine B, Axelrod BN. Determining an appropriate cutting score for indication of impairment on the Montreal Cognitive Assessment. *Int J Geriatr Psychiatry* 2012;**27** (11):1189–1194.

30. Burton L, Tyson SF. Screening for cognitive impairment after stroke: a systematic review of psychometric properties and clinical utility. *J Rehab Med.* 2015;**47**(3):193–203.

31. Dubois B, Slachevsky A, Litvan I, et al. The FAB: a Frontal Assessment Battery at bedside. *Neurology.* 2000;**55** (11):1621–1626.

32. Ylikoski R, Jokinen H, Andersen P, et al. Comparison of the Alzheimer's Disease Assessment Scale Cognitive Subscale and the Vascular Dementia Assessment Scale in differentiating elderly individuals with different degrees of white matter changes. The LADIS Study. *Dementand Geriatr Cogn Disord.* 2007;**24** (2):73–81.

33. Folstein MF, Folstein SE, McHugh PR. "Mini-mental state": a practical method for grading the cognitive state of patients for the clinician. *J Psychiatr Res.* 1975;**12** (3):189–198.

34. Pendlebury ST, Cuthbertson FC, Welch SJ, et al. Underestimation of cognitive impairment by Mini-Mental State Examination versus the Montreal Cognitive Assessment in patients with transient ischemic attack and stroke: a population-based study. *Stroke.* 2010;**41** (6):1290–1293.

35. Smith EE, Schneider JA, Wardlaw JM, et al. Cerebral microinfarcts: the invisible lesions. *Lancet Neurol.* 2012;**11** (3):272–282.

36. Tatemichi TK, Desmond DW, Prohovnik I. Strategic infarcts in vascular dementia: a clinical and brain imaging experience. *Arzneimittel-Forschung.* 1995;**45**(3A):371–385.

37. Wardlaw JM, Smith EE, Biessels GJ, et al. Neuroimaging standards for research into small vessel disease and its contribution to ageing and neurodegeneration. *Lancet Neurol.* 2013;**12**(8):822–838.

38. Pullicino PM, Miller LL, Alexandrov AV, et al. Infraputaminal "Lacunes": clinical and pathological correlations. *Stroke.* 1995;**26**(9):1598–1602.

39. Das RR, Seshadri S, Beiser AS, et al. Prevalence and correlates of silent cerebral infarcts in the Framingham offspring study. *Stroke.* 2008;**39**(11):2929–2935.

40. Vermeer SE, Prins ND, den Heijer T, et al. Silent brain infarcts and the risk of dementia and cognitive decline. *N Engl J Med.* 2003;**348**(13):1215–1222.

41. Debette S, Markus HS. The clinical importance of white matter hyperintensities on brain magnetic resonance imaging: systematic review and meta-analysis. *BMJ.* 2010;**341**:c3666.

42. Wardlaw JM, Valdes Hernandez MC, Munoz-Maniega S. What are white matter hyperintensities made of? Relevance to vascular cognitive impairment. *J Am Heart Assoc.* 2015;**4**(6):001140.

43. Greenberg SM, Vernooij MW, Cordonnier C, et al. Cerebral microbleeds: a guide to detection and interpretation. *Lancet Neurol.* 2009;**8**(2):165–174.

44. Fein G, Di Sclafani V, Tanabe J, et al. Hippocampal and cortical atrophy predict dementia in subcortical ischemic vascular disease. *Neurology.* 2000;**55**(11):1626–1635.

45. Jokinen H, Lipsanen J, Schmidt R, et al. Brain atrophy accelerates cognitive decline in cerebral small vessel disease: the LADIS study. *Neurology.* 2012;**78**(22):1785–1792.

46. Johnson KA, Gregas M, Becker JA, et al. Imaging of amyloid burden and distribution in cerebral amyloid angiopathy. *Ann Neurol.* 2007;**62**(3):229–234.

47. Mattsson N, Zetterberg H, Hansson O, et al. CSF biomarkers and incipient Alzheimer disease in patients with mild cognitive impairment. *JAMA.* 2009;**302**(4):385–393.

48. Vilar-Bergua A, Riba-Llena I, Nafria C, et al. Blood and CSF biomarkers in brain subcortical ischemic vascular disease: involved pathways and clinical applicability. *J Cereb Blood Flow Metab.* 2016;**36**(1):55–71.

49. Huisa BN, Rosenberg GA. Binswanger's disease: toward a diagnosis agreement and therapeutic approach. *Expert Rev Neurotherapeutics.* 2014;**14**(10):1203–1213.

50. American Psychiatric Association. *Diagnostic and Statistical Manual of Mental Disorders.* 3rd ed. Washington, D.C.: American Psychiatric Association, 1987.

51. American Psychiatric Association. *Diagnostic and Statistical Manual of Mental Disorders.* 4th ed. Washington, DC: American Psychiatric Association, 1994.

52. Chui HC, Mack W, Jackson JE, et al. Clinical criteria for the diagnosis of vascular dementia: a multicenter study of comparability and interrater reliability. *Arch Neurol.* 2000;**57**(2):191–196.

53. Roman GC, Tatemichi TK, Erkinjuntti T, et al. Vascular dementia: diagnostic criteria for research studies. Report of the NINDS-AIREN International Workshop. *Neurology.* 1993;**43**(2):250–260.

54. Organization WH. *The ICD-10 Classification of Mental and Behavioral Disorders: Diagnostic Criteria for Research.* Geneva: World Health Organization, 1993.

55. American Psychiatric Association. *Diagnostic and Statistical Manual of Mental Disorders*. 5th ed.: American Psychiatric Association, 2013.

56. Tripathi M, Vibha D. Reversible dementia. *Indian J Psychiatry*. 2009;**51**(Suppl. 1): S52–55.

57. Wright CB, Flores A. Vascular contributions to cognitive impairment. *Neurol Clin Pract*. 2015;5(3):201–208.

58. Merino JG, Warach S. Imaging of acute stroke. *Nature Revs Neurol*. 2010;**6** (10):560–571.

The Brain at Risk Stage

Mahmoud Reza Azarpazhooh and Vladimir Hachinski

Resist beginnings; too late is the medicine prepared when the disease has gained strength by long delays.
Ovid, Roman Poet, 43 BC–18 AD

Introduction

The brain at risk stage represents the stage when someone remains symptomless, but has risk factors.[1] The prevalence cannot be ascertained precisely, but almost certainly, asymptomatic individuals largely exceed the number of symptomatic individuals. A better understanding of this stage is vital as the early identification of those at risk provides the opportunity for therapeutic interventions and preventive measures.[2] However, such an approach needs a dramatic change in our philosophy of health care delivery: from a passive diagnosis of dementia and symptomatic treatment of frank symptoms to active multidisciplinary identification of mild cognitive impairment and even a stage prior to this – brain-at-risk with prevention of dementia and stroke simultaneously.[3]

Joint Prevention of Stroke and Dementia

Epidemiological Evidence

The Canadian Study in Health and Aging found that if persons over the age of 65 years or older had a stroke, 64 percent of them had some cognitive impairment. Conversely, among individuals who had some cognitive impairment, 25 percent had had a stroke. Thus epidemiologic evidence suggests that stroke and dementia pose risks for each other.[4]

The REGARD Study followed over 23,000 individuals for over 6 years and cognitive determinations were done each year. Over that period, 515 individuals had a stroke. Not surprisingly, this was associated with cognitive impairment. However, what is novel about this study is that researchers had information about the pre-stroke cognitive status. They found that after a stroke, the slope of cognitive decline became steeper, especially of executive function, suggesting that the stroke had triggered an ongoing process.[5] It is likely that this was an interaction between Alzheimer and cerebrovascular pathology. The commonest outcome of cerebrovascular disease is not a clinical stroke, but cognitive impairment. In the Rotterdam Study, for each clinical stroke there were 5 so called silent strokes that resulted in subtle neurological signs, decreases in processing speed and also executive function (Figure 3.1).[6]

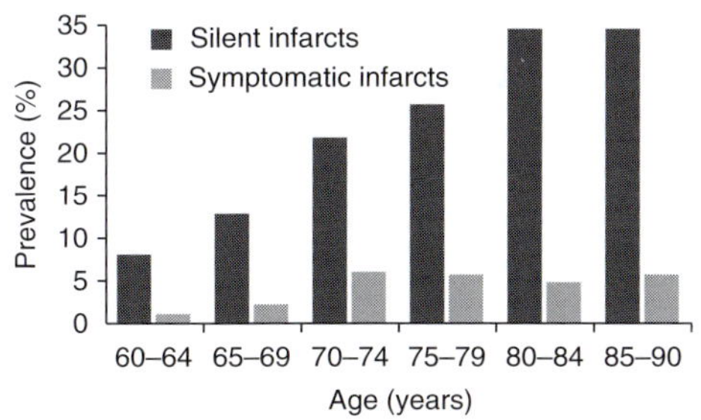

Figure 3.1 Prevalence of infarcts in the Rotterdam Scan Study.
(Adapted from Vermeer SE et al. *NEJM* 2003. 348: 1215–1222)[6]

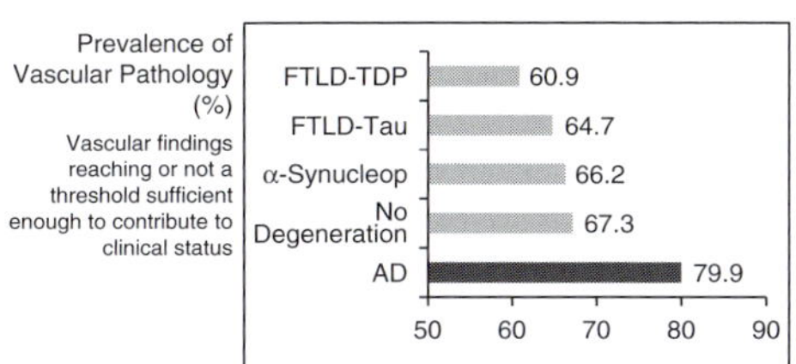

Figure 3.2 Contribution of cerebrovascular disease in autopsy-confirmed neurogenerative disease cases. National Alzheimer's Coordinating Center Database 6205 autopsy cases.
Toledo JB, Arnold SE, Raible K, Brettschneider J, Xie SX, Grossman M, Monsell SE et al. Contribution of cerebrovascular disease in autopsy confirmed neurodegenerative disease cases in the National Alzheimer's Coordinating Centre. *Brain.* 2013;136(pt 9):2697–2706.

Most Alzheimer pathology (plaques and tangles) occur silently without resulting in cognitive impairment. However, if an individual has neurodegenerative pathology and a vascular component, this doubles the chances that they will manifest dementia.

The clinical evidence for an interaction has long been recognized. Reports from three continents suggest that at least a quarter of stroke patients have significant cognitive impairment at three months.[7]

Among the clinicopathological evidence for interaction the most compelling comes from the Nun's Study. Only 57 percent of the nuns who had a pathological diagnosis of Alzheimer disease had any cognitive difficulty in life. However, if in addition they had a cortical infarct, then 75 percent of them did, and if they had one of more deep small infarcts, then 93 percent of them exhibited cognitive problems.[8]

This suggests that Alzheimer and cerebrovascular pathology interact. Experimentally, a cerebral infarct in the presence of brain amyloid (a model of Alzheimer disease) becomes larger and grows compared to infarcts induced to control animals, and the inflammation is greater and it festers, compared to settling down as occurs in control animals. This suggests that a stroke may exacerbate the consequences of amyloid deposits by creating a malignant triangle of ischemia, inflammation, and amyloid deposition.[9]

Prevention Strategies

Nonpharmacological managements

Physical activity

Physical, mental, and social exercise seems to be the combination that most effectively can protect against stroke and Alzheimer disease. Growing evidence suggests that physical activity at the recommended level, namely 30 minutes of moderate exercise at least 5 times a week has great beneficial effect on overall health and also mounting evidence that there is also a more direct effect on the brain. The attributable risk of physical inactivity in the Canadian population was higher than any other risk factors, including hypertension;[10] i.e., physical inactivity is not as strong a risk factor as hypertension, but involves a larger number of individuals. Although the best protective association was observed in dementia with vascular components, physical activity may also decrease the incidence of Alzheimer disease.[11,12] Even patients with underlying cognitive impairment may still benefit from physical activities.[13]

Cognitive Activity and Brain Reserve

In terms of mental exercise, it is uncertain whether the association with intellectual activity and preservation is cause or consequence of brain health. Those inclined to exercise their minds are probably in better shape than those who do not. Nevertheless, no harm ensues from doing puzzles or other intellectual activity that is stimulating. Exercising the mind in a particular skill will improve that skill, but there is no evidence that acquiring one skill will enhance others. For example, doing puzzles will enhance the ability to solve them; however, this ability does not easily translate into enhancing other intellectual abilities. Even though they might be confounded by several socioeconomic variables, many studies have shown that those with a higher level of cognitive activity, for example education and bilingualism, are at a lower risk of dementia than their counterparts. This led to the concept of "brain reserve." In this theory, a possible protective effect cognitive exercise might be due to a more efficient neural network with a greater capacity or the possibility of better compensation after a network disruption.[14–16]

Social Engagement and Cognitive Leisure Activities

Social engagements, be it visiting friends and colleagues or going to charity events, and cognitive leisure activities are protective factors against dementia.[17–19] While the reasons of such a protective effect are not clear, people with more social engagement may have a wider neural network (brain reserve theory) or may have a better understanding of dementia symptoms, and its preventive measuring via sharing knowledge with friends and relatives in their frequent interactions. Although this theory might be confounded by the fact that people with dementia or major mental conditions, such as depression, may decrease their social activities, there is no harm to recommend social engagements and cognitive leisure activities to the public.

Depression

Many studies have shown a strong association between depression, particularly in the elderly, and cognitive impairment.[20,21] The prevalence of depression is higher in dementia with vascular components and mixed subtypes as compared to Alzheimer disease.[22] One important unanswered question is whether or not depression follows, coincides with, or precedes dementia. Nevertheless, screening, identification, and appropriate diagnosis of depression are highly recommended in any clinical/research setting of dementia.

Diet

Some studies showed that a healthy diet may decrease the risk of dementia and stroke. A healthy diet, such as the Mediterranean diet, probably would go a long way in achieving a healthy lifestyle and moderating whatever risks the patient may bear. Logically, major vascular risk factors, such as diabetes, hyperlipidemia, and hypertension may be prevented or modified by healthy diet. In addition, a diet high in antioxidant nutrients, such as vitamins E and C, carotenoids, flavonoids, and enzymatic cofactors may reduce inflammation and consequently can affect the chance of dementia.[23] On the other hand, the modern rapid food diet typically comes replete with calories, full of unsaturated fats and loaded with salt. All of these have consequences. The calories contribute to the obesity epidemic, unsaturated fats promote atherosclerosis, and salt contributes to increasing blood pressure. One particularly insidious form of calorie intake is by sugared drinks. They are usually sweetened with fructose that has no natural feedback mechanism in the brain. This means that individuals can continue to drink these sweet drinks without feeling satiated. By contrast, products sweetened with sucrose, have a natural feedback mechanism in the human brain. Individuals at liberty to drink sugar drinks as they wish put on weight whereas persons consuming candy at will did not.

Tobacco

Tobacco is well recognized as a risk factor for all types of stroke, and now it is evident that it is also a risk factor for Alzheimer disease, including second-hand smoke. The hazardous effects might be explained by a combination of cerebral perfusion reduction, stroke, accelerated cerebral atrophy, damage to the blood brain barrier, and white matter lesions.[24]

Alcohol

Alcohol in excess of the recommended dose – two standard drinks per day for a man and one to two drinks for a woman – increases the risk of stroke and Alzheimer disease.

A standard drink is a 5 ounces (150 ml) glass of wine, 12 ounces of beer, or 1.5 ounces of liquor. Although in these amounts, alcohol may have protective effects, but for each person who benefits, many more are harmed.

Alcohol in moderation has been shown to be associated with decreased risk of stroke and dementia.[25] Although arguments have been made for particular types of wine or drink being best, it is alcohol itself that has a modest generic protective effect. Alcohol probably should never be recommended for brain protection. If someone has the urge to have a drink, they should go for a hike and take a friend.

Sleep

Sleep disorders and dementia (including Alzheimer disease) may have a casual interactive association. Although sleep problems might be a consequence of dementia, some studies showed that poor sleep is a modifiable risk factor for dementia and Alzheimer disease.[26–29] Similar to other joint risk factors, sleep disorders might be a risk factor for vascular disorders.

Vascular Risk Factors Reduction

Since stroke and Alzheimer disease share the main risk factors, it behooves us to address not only whether the cerebrovascular and Alzheimer pathologies coexist, but also whether they interact. It is also encouraging that the main modifiable risk factors for stroke are the same as for Alzheimer disease.

In addition to this list, now it is clear that atrial fibrillation also represents a risk for both dementia, including Alzheimer disease[30] and for stroke, and it is highly treatable.

Table 3.1 Main proposed risk and protective factors common for stroke and dementia

Nonmodifiable Risk Factors	Risk Factors	Protective Factors
Advanced age	Cerebrovascular disease/stroke	High education
Genetic factors (Apo E4)	Cardiovascular diseases	Physical activity
Family history	Hypertension	Antihypertensives
	Hypercholesterolemia	Statins
	Obesity	Active lifestyle
	Diabetes	Mediterranean diet (added)
	Smoking	
	Homocysteine	
	Stress	
	Depression	
	Atrial fibrillation (added)	Anticoagulation (added)

(Modified from Soloman A et al. JIM 2014)

Hypertension

Hypertension is the single most powerful and treatable risk factor both for stroke and for dementia, that applies to both systolic and diastolic blood pressures.[31] The relationship is quite clear in early and midlife, and it becomes less so towards the later stages of life. This is probably due to the fact that in a population the systolic blood pressure tends to go up with age and eventually declines. Diastolic blood pressure increases up to a point then also declines. A number of studies have found a direct relationship between blood pressure and cognition preservation and hence ill grounded speculations that hypertension should not be treated in the elderly.[32] One reason for this relationship may be that when an Alzheimer process infiltrates the insula, a key center for cardiovascular control, the blood pressure tends to drop.[33] Another contributing factor may be that with age there is an increase in pulse pressure. This type of perfusion of the brain may make it less optimal than when the systolic and diastolic blood pressures are closer together.[34] Hypertension should be treated at all ages.

Atrial Fibrillation

Atrial fibrillation puts the individuals at a risk of stroke an average of 5 percent per year. More recently it has also shown that it also represents a risk factor for cognitive impairment.[35–37] Luckily warfarin has been available since 1948 and more recently new anticoagulants that target factor X are easier to take and have fewer interactions with food than warfarin, but on the other hand it is not yet certain how to stop bleeding with these new anticoagulants. It is probably only a question of time before such measures are discovered.

Diabetes

Diabetes has a reciprocal cause and effect relation with cognitive decline. Diabetes may lead to dementia via a range of mechanisms, including vascular lesions,[38] activation of microglia and peripheral and central inflammatory response,[39] and blood brain barrier disruption. In addition, neurodegenerative brain lesion, such as amyloid deposition especially in the hypothalamus,[40] may cause central insulin resistance. Such a bidirectional relationship emphasizes the importance of diabetes prevention in joint management of stroke and dementia.

Hyperlipidemia

Several studies showed that hyperlipidemia is a major risk factor for stroke. Recently, a significant decline in the incidence of stroke in high-income countries is partially due to better prevention of vascular risk factors, including hyperlipidemia and widespread use of statins. Theoretically, by controlling stroke we may expect that statins can decrease the chance of dementia; however, the results of current studies are inconsistent, and this effect is still debatable. Nevertheless, statins have become a part of best practice to prevent vascular disorders.

Homocysteine

High homocysteine levels have been associated with increased risk of stroke and dementia.[41] What is less clear is whether treatment of homocysteine makes a difference to the risk.[42]

Inflammation

Inflammation as manifested in infections and chronic inflammatory states reflected in the CRP represents a risk factor for both stroke and Alzheimer disease. Again, it is not certain that treating the inflammatory marker makes a difference to the outcomes.

Hormone Replacement Therapy

The risk of developing Alzheimer disease increases in postmenopausal women.[43] The results of studies assessing the risks and benefit of hormone replacement therapy on Alzheimer disease are inconsistent.[44] A meta-analysis of four studies in participants with a wide range of dementia severity found some beneficial effect from estrogen on cognition. Some studies showed that estrogen therapy may improve cognitive functions in recently menopausal women.[45] According to Women's Health Initiative (WHI) study, for postmenopausal women aged 65 years or older estrogen plus progestin therapy did not prevent mild cognitive impairment.[43] Despite the lack of randomized trials, it is possible that timing has significant effects on the possible effects of hormone therapy.[46] Based on current information, the risks of hormone replacement therapies with estrogen and progesterone outweigh the possible benefits.

The Genetic Brackets

A person may well ask "What if I have the wrong genes, for example, the *APOE-4* allele? What good would it do to restrict myself and control all these risk factors when in the end I end up with the wrong outcome?" It turns out that the presence of *APOE-4* magnifies the risk of developing dementia considerably, but by the same token treatment of the risk factors, decreases that risk in proportion to the heightened hazard.

Adjusted RR Subjects with normal and ε4 – as reference	Antihypertensive therapy	
	Yes	No
Midlife high BP/ε4–	1.5 (0.8–2.4)	2.4 (0.6–10.4)
Midlife high BP/ε4+	1.9 (0.7–4.5)	10.8 (1.4–83.5)

Figure 3.3 The Honolulu Aging Study. APOE, ε4, midlife BPL and antihypertensives.

There is also suggestive evidence that risk factors such as alcohol intake and physical inactivity are also associated with a magnified effect of *APOE-4*. Probably the reduction may result in a proportionate decrease in the risk.

Enhancing Prevention

Urbanization and westernization have revolutionized lifestyles worldwide. It is difficult to keep a healthy lifestyle in an unhealthy environment. Automation, decreased need for physical activity, and crowded cities do not encourage physical activity; the air is polluted and so is the environment by many outlets that allow us to consume fast foods at low prices everywhere. The message is for increased consumption, multiplied many times by direct and subtle advertising. The new world opened by the internet and social media again foster multiple brief interactions that paradoxically may breed indolence and isolation amidst a surfeit of superficial communication. If prevention is to be enhanced at the brain at risk stage, the approach has to be at multiple levels.

International

In September of 2011, the UN adopted a resolution[47] addressing the rising threat of non-communicable diseases, now accounting for about 60 percent of the disease burden, particularly in middle- and low-income countries. The United Nations has targeted cardiovascular disease (heart disease and stroke, cancer, pulmonary disease and diabetes), all of which share the risk factors of physical inactivity, unhealthy diet, tobacco, and alcohol consumption.

The World Health Organization and national governments are trying to implement the recommendations, and as physicians we have a special role to play to make sure that these decisions become reality.

The Community

The community also has a large role to play, since many of our lives are shaped by where we live. The family continues to have an important role, particularly in teaching children healthy lifestyle habits.

The Individual

Last and most important, there is the individual. In asking an individual to control risk factors, we are addressing the challenge of changing human behavior, a notoriously difficult task. However, it is well established that the most powerful agent in changing human behavior is another interested human being. Some successful examples are Alcoholics Anonymous and other venues in which the individual works with another interested individual. There are ongoing studies evaluating this approach, and there are also a number of virtual versions of this, be it online programs that allow interaction with the individual or increasingly with smartphones that may individualize messages to the individual and if necessary, give the individual access to another person. An African proverb states: "If you want to go fast, go alone. If you want to go far, go together." Prevention is a long road.

The ideal is to control the risk factors and the brain at risk stage, but it is never too late, although earlier is better.

Summary

The prevention of stroke and dementia need a comprehensive joint program. This model should include a multidisciplinary approach controlling risk factors in symptomatic patients or ideally in those at risk yet still asymptomatic: the brain at risk stage.

References

1. Hachinski V. Preventable senility: a call for action against the vascular dementias. *Lancet*. 1992; **12**(340):645–648.

2. Hachinski V. Vascular cognitive impairment: a unified approach to cognitive disorders. *Brain and Cognition*. 2007;**63**:196–255.

3. Bowler JV, Steenhuis R, Hachinski V. Conceptual background to vascular cognitive impairment. *Alzheimer Dis Assoc Disord*. 1999 Dec 1 [cited 1999 Dec 1];**13** (Supplement 3).

4. Jin Y-P, Di Legge S, Østbye T, Feightner JW, Saposnik G, Hachinski V. Is stroke history reliably reported by elderly with cognitive impairment? A community-based study. *Neuroepidemiology*. 2010;**35**:215–220.

5. Levine DA, Galecki AT, Langa KM, et al. Trajectory of cognitive decline after incident stroke. *JAMA*. 2015;**314**:41–51.

6. Vermeer SE, Prins ND, den Heijer T, Hofman A, Koudstaal PJ, Breteler MMB. Silent brain infarcts and the risk of dementia and cognitive decline. *N Engl J Med*. 2001;**348**:1215–1222.

7. Pendlebury ST, Rothwell PM. Prevalence, incidence, and factors associated with pre-stroke and post-stroke dementia: a systematic review and meta-analysis. *Lancet Neurol*. 2009;**8**:1006–1018.

8. Snowdon DA, Greiner LH, Mortimer JA, Riley KP, Greiner PA, Markesbery WR. Brain infarction and the clinical expression of Alzheimer disease: The Nun Study. *JAMA*. 1997;**277**:813–817.

9. Thiel A, Cechetto DF, Heiss W-D, Hachinski V, Whitehead SN. Amyloid burden, neuroinflammation, and links to cognitive decline after ischemic stroke. *Stroke*. 2014;**45**:2825–2829.

10. Young TK, Hachinski V. The population approach to stroke prevention: a Canadian perspective. *Clin Invest Med, Médecine Clinique et Experimentale* 2003;**26**:78–86.

11. Rockwood K, Middleton L. Physical activity and the maintenance of cognitive function. *Alzheimer's Dement*. 2007;3(2 Suppl):S38–44.

12. Ravaglia G, Forti P, Lucicesare A, et al. Physical activity and dementia risk in the elderly: findings from a prospective Italian study. *Neurology*. 2008;**70**:1786–1794.

13. Lautenschlager NT, Cox KL, Flicker L, et al. Effect of physical activity on cognitive function in older adults at risk for Alzheimer disease: a randomized trial. *JAMA*. 2008;**300**:1027–1037.

14. Stern Y. Cognitive reserve and Alzheimer disease. *Alzheimer Dis Assoc Disord*. 2006;**20**:112–117.

15. Roe CM, Xiong C, Miller JP, Morris JC. Education and Alzheimer disease without dementia: support for the cognitive reserve hypothesis. *Neurology.* 2007;**68**:223–228.

16. Craik FIM, Bialystok E, Freedman M. Delaying the onset of Alzheimer disease: bilingualism as a form of cognitive reserve. *Neurology.* 2010;**75**(19):1726–1729.

17. Fratiglioni L, Wang H-X. Brain reserve hypothesis in dementia. *J Alzheimer's Dis.* 2007;**12**(1):11–22.

18. Kang H. Correlates of social engagement in nursing home residents with dementia. *Asian Nurs Res.* 2012;**6**(2):75–81.

19. Stern C, Munn Z. Cognitive leisure activities and their role in preventing dementia: a systematic review. *JBI Lib Systematic Revs.* 2007;7(29): 1292–1332.

20. Steffens DC, Otey E, Alexopoulos GS, et al. Perspectives on depression, mild cognitive impairment, and cognitive decline. *Arch Gen Psych.* 2006;**63**(2):130–138.

21. Tsuno N, Homma A. What is the association between depression and Alzheimer's disease? *Expert Rev Neurotherapeutics.* 2009;**9**(11):1667–1676.

22. Castilla-Puentes RC, Habeych ME. Subtypes of depression among patients with Alzheimer's disease and other dementias. *Alzheimer's Dement.* 2010;**6**(1):63–69.

23. Gillette Guyonnet S, Abellan Van Kan G, Andrieu S, et al. IANA task force on nutrition and cognitive decline with aging. *J Nutri Health Aging.* 2007;**11**(2): 132–152.

24. Peters R. Blood pressure, smoking and alcohol use, association with vascular dementia. *Exp Gerontol.* 2012;**47**(11):865–872.

25. Peters R, Peters J, Warner J, Beckett N, Bulpitt C. Alcohol, dementia and cognitive decline in the elderly: a systematic review. *Age Ageing.* 2008;**37**(5):505–512.

26. Spira AP, Chen-Edinboro LP, Wu MN, Yaffe K. Impact of sleep on the risk of cognitive decline and dementia. *Curr Opin Psychiatry.* 2014;**27**(6):478–483.

27. Lal C, Strange C, Bachman D. Neurocognitive impairment in obstructive sleep apnea. *Chest.* 2012;**141**(6):1601–1610.

28. Garcia S, Gunstad J. Sleep and physical activity as modifiable risk factors in age-associated cognitive decline. *Sleep Biologic Rhythms.* 2015;**14**(1):3–11.

29. Lim ASP, Kowgier M, Yu L, Buchman AS, Bennett DA. Sleep fragmentation and the risk of incident Alzheimer's disease and cognitive decline in older persons. *Sleep.* 2013;**36**:1027–1032.

30. Dublin S, Anderson ML, Haneuse SJ, et al. Atrial fibrillation and risk of dementia: a prospective cohort study. *J Am Geriatr Soc.* 2011;**59**(8):1369–1375.

31. Skoog I, Gustafson D. Update on hypertension and Alzheimer's disease. *Neurologic Res.* 2006;**28**(6):605–611.

32. Sörös P, Hachinski V. Cardiovascular and neurological causes of sudden death after ischaemic stroke. *Lancet Neurology.* 2012;**11**(2):179–188.

33. Royall DR, Gao J-H, Kellogg DL. Insular Alzheimer's disease pathology as a cause of "age-related" autonomic dysfunction and mortality in the non-demented elderly. *Med Hypotheses.* 2006;**67**(4):747–758.

34. Wardlaw JM, Chappell FM, Valdés Hernández MDC, et al. White matter hyperintensity reduction and outcomes after minor stroke. *Neurology.* 2017;**89**(10):1003–1010.

35. Baidac G, Petrescu A, Sterea A, Spiru L. Correlation between atrial fibrillation, stroke and dementia. *Alzheimer's & Dementia.* 2011;7(4):S369–S370.

36. Shah AD, Merchant FM, Delurgio DB. Atrial fibrillation and risk of dementia/cognitive decline. *J Atrial Fibrillation.* 2016;8(5):1353.

37. Jurašić M-J, Morović S, Antić S, Zavoreo I, Demarin V. Stroke and Dementia in Atrial Fibrillation. In: Atrial Fibrillation – Basic Research and Clinical Applications. InTech; 2012 [cited 2012 Jan 11].

38. Gorelick PB, Scuteri A, Black SE, et al. Vascular contributions to cognitive impairment and dementia: a statement for

healthcare professionals from the American Heart Association / American Stroke Association. *Stroke*. 2011;**42**(9):2672–2713.

39. Dey A, Hao S, Erion JR, Wosiski-Kuhn M, Stranahan AM. Glucocorticoid sensitization of microglia in a genetic mouse model of obesity and diabetes. *J Neuroimmunol*. 2014;**269**(1–2):20–27.

40. Ishii M, Iadecola C. Metabolic and non-cognitive manifestations of Alzheimer's disease: the hypothalamus as both culprit and target of pathology. *Cell Metabol*. 2015;**22**(5):761–776.

41. Spence JD, Yi Q, Hankey GJ. B vitamins in stroke prevention: time to reconsider. *Lancet Neurol*. 2017;**16**(9):750–760.

42. Finsterer J. Low risk of ischaemic stroke in hyperhomocysteinaemia. *Lancet Neurol*. 2017;**16**(9):682–683.

43. Shumaker SA, Legault C, Rapp SR, et al. Estrogen plus progestin and the incidence of dementia and mild cognitive impairment in postmenopausal women: The Women's Health Initiative Memory Study: a randomized controlled trial. *JAMA*. 2003;**289**(20):2663–2673.

44. Manson JE, Chlebowski RT, Stefanick ML, et al. Menopausal hormone therapy and health outcomes during the intervention and extended poststopping phases of The Women's Health Initiative randomized trials. *ObstetGynecol Sur*. 2014;**69**(2):83–85.

45. Yaffe K, Sawaya G, Lieberburg I, Grady D. Estrogen therapy in postmenopausal women: effects on cognitive function and dementia. *JAMA*. 1998;**279**(9):688–695.

46. Lobo RA. Where are we 10 years after the Women's Health Initiative? *J Clin Endocrinol Metab*. 2013;**98**(5):1771–1780.

47. UN Department of Economic and Social Affairs and Population Division. *World urbanization prospects: The 2014 revision, highlights*. New York, NY: United Nations, 2014.

Chapter 4

The Patient with Cognitive Impairment

Krister Håkansson, Tiia Ngandu, and Miia Kivipelto

Introduction

In this chapter we will describe persons with cognitive impairment: different types of impairments and different interventions to counteract – or even reverse – continued cognitive worsening. We will take a clinical case as a starting point to illustrate the complexities involved in the clinical evaluation of a person with cognitive impairment and the risk of diagnostic errors, a case that summarizes much of what this chapter is about. From there, we move on to describe variability in cognitive trajectories in old age, both in normal aging and when cognitive impairment occurs. The part about dementia will focus on the most common type of dementia, Alzheimer disease, but also emphasizing how neuropathological and vascular components typically combine and contribute to different degrees in the clinical picture. In the diagnostic procedure we describe, we emphasize the need to establish whether a cognitive decline has preceded the visit to the physician or not, and we also include a suggested step-by-step procedure for the clinical evaluation. We then move on to the question if cognitive impairment can be prevented or delayed through nonpharmacological strategies. Methodological challenges in epidemiological association studies include consideration of the long and progressive subclinical phase that precedes a clinical diagnosis. This has raised doubts whether factors associated with subsequent cognitive impairment in these studies can be translated into effective nonpharmacological interventions. We summarize the evidence that exists for candidate intervention factors from previous observational association studies, and in addition shortly review results from studies that have based interventions on some of these factors. As many different factors have showed associations with subsequent cognitive impairment, we discuss the possibility that multimodal intervention strategies may be a more promising approach. We finally evaluate the evidence from three existing multimodal intervention studies and discuss implications for future developments of this field.

The Person behind the Diagnosis

Emma is 87 years old, used to teach literature at a university, and is still an intelligent person in many ways, in spite of a stroke eight years ago in the lower part of left frontotemporal area, a damage to her brain that still affects mobility in her right arm and with a remaining slur in her speech, in spite of a remarkable recovery. Emma was also diagnosed with possible Alzheimer disease (AD) two years ago, largely based on emerging problems in her episodic memory, both confirmed by her subjective complaints and by a score of "only" 24 on the MMSE, a level perceived to reflect considerable decline in the light of her previous performance as a well-respected and successful academic. This diagnosis was also supported by a MRI scan showing considerable atrophy in both the medial temporal lobe and in both lateral ventricles.

Taken together, these features suggest that Emma is a person with possible Alzheimer dementia with probable vascular involvement. Her history can also make us think that a large brain reserve up to now has enabled her to resist a substantial pathological influence on her cognitive function. We can suspect that the preceding stroke may both have contributed to elicit the progressive AD pathology[1] and to have added components of cognitive impairments atypical to AD (see Chapter 5). These impairments may not only be due to the stroke itself and the brain areas directly affected by it, but also to suboptimal vascular functioning that constituted a risk factor for the stroke, for the development of dementia, and furthermore for other vascular damage with cognitive consequences. As no cognitive tests were conducted after the stroke, we know little about when and how the cognitive impairment started that preceded the present clinical picture.

Emma's problems are in many ways typical for an old person with cognitive impairment; she probably suffers from AD, the most common type of dementia, possibly mixed with cognitive impairment of a vascular origin. This addition of a vascular component is common and adds to the complexity of the clinical picture, compared to pure AD. But Emma is also a unique person with characteristics that affect the clinical presentation of the disease. Other chapters in this book illustrate the heterogeneity of symptoms in vascular cognitive impairment, which necessitates an open attitude when such a patient is encountered. Vascular brain damage can occur in different locations and magnitudes, including mini-strokes and lacunar strokes that in the case of "silent infarcts" may even have gone unnoticed by the patient (see Chapter 5); it can have a rather specific localization in the brain, and the cognitive and behavioral problems will consequently be related to the specific function; or it could be widely distributed and then more probably cause a general impairment in a variety of functions and in slower cognitive processing in addition. Thus, in contrast to damages caused by several other dementing disorders, damages caused by vascular insufficiencies give rise to behavioral and cognitive changes that can be relatively nonpredictable and difficult to detect in routine examination. Many of the screening instruments used by general practicioners and in memory clinics (e.g., MMSE) are also relatively insensitive for vascular types of cognitive impairment.

There are other reasons for openness when we encounter a person with possible cognitive problems as this person often has reached a mature age as aging itself introduces increased heterogeneity (see Chapter 1). This principle of increasing heterogeneity with advanced age not only applies to the level of cognitive performance within age cohorts, but also to differences in cognitive aging trajectories over time. This means that some persons maintain most of their cognitive capacity even in old age, while others, in spite of non-existent or few neuropathologies, may show a more pronounced decline. The only cognitive domain that seems to be universally affected to at least some degree by aging, even when birth cohort effects on both cognitive levels and trajectories are taken into account, is cognitive speed, e.g., perceptual speed and executive speed.[2] For cognitively well-preserved old persons, we can thus expect that their performance will be similar to that of younger persons – especially if they are given some extra time to perform these tasks. Besides aging-related processes and dementia-related pathology, other factors such as previous life exposures, birth cohort effects,[3] and personality traits may affect the clinical presentation.

The clinical evaluation is furthermore complicated by another type of variability; that the same person may vary in performance levels between different occasions, i.e., intra-individual variability. It has been shown that the tendency to show this kind of day-to-day variation may be more typical for some individuals than for others[4,5] and in addition more pronounced in persons with dementia, compared to cognitively intact persons of the same age[6] (see also Chapter 1).

There are probably few medical conditions that are more complex to evaluate than cognitive impairment. In clinical evaluations, we normally follow the routine examination and tests and sometimes rely on cognitive short cuts and make decisions faster than we should (e.g., not evaluating cognitive functioning), resulting in "premature closure."[7] Premature closure means that we base our decisions on fewer considerations than we should. A specific risk with premature closure is that diagnostic efforts may stop when a certain disease has been identified, also when that disease is mixed with other diseases with less salient symptoms, i.e., in cases of comorbidity[8] (e.g., vascular components in persons who fulfill diagnostic criteria of AD – or vice versa).

Persons with Cognitive Impairment

When people come to a memory clinic, they usually have cognitive complaints that some-times can become verified through neuropsychological testing. In the case that no such verification can be made, the person can be classified to have subjective cognitive impair-ment (SCI). Even if diagnostic criteria are not fulfilled for objective cognitive impairment, these patients on average perform somewhat poorer on cognitive tests and the risk of further cognitive impairment and dementia and AD is higher compared to persons without these complaints.[9] Psychiatric and behavioral problems such as depression, burn out, and stress are common contributing factors for SCI but can also be risk factors or predictors of further dementia development.

A dementia diagnosis is usually preceded by a long period of subclinical neuropatholo-gical deterioration, with mild cognitive impairment (MCI), or mild neurocognitive disorder in the new DSM-V,[10] as a transition phase before diagnostic criteria for dementia have been reached. Based on such a trajectory of progressive cognitive decline leading up to dementia, it has been suggested that SCI should be considered as a pre-MCI stage, which in turn can be considered as a stage of pre-dementia.[11] One problem with this assumption is that there are no generally accepted diagnostic criteria for SCI. Possibly as a result, the reported SCI prevalence shows a large variation between different 65+ populations, according to one review from 25 percent to 56 percent[12] although part of this variation may also have been caused by differences in sample selection between different studies.[12] Data from two memory clinics also showed dramatic differences in prevalence of SCI among their patients, 7.5 percent in one case and 38 percent in the other,[9] possibly due to similar reasons as in the population-based studies.

Second, even if many persons with either SCI or MCI may progress in cognitive impairment and eventually be diagnosed with dementia, this is not the case for all. Some are stable, and some regress to levels of cognitive performance that are normal for their age.[13,14]

Of critical importance when evaluating a person with cognitive complaints is recogni-tion of the normal variation in cognitive performance among elderly healthy individuals. Differences in intelligence and in various lifetime exposures all contribute to differences in

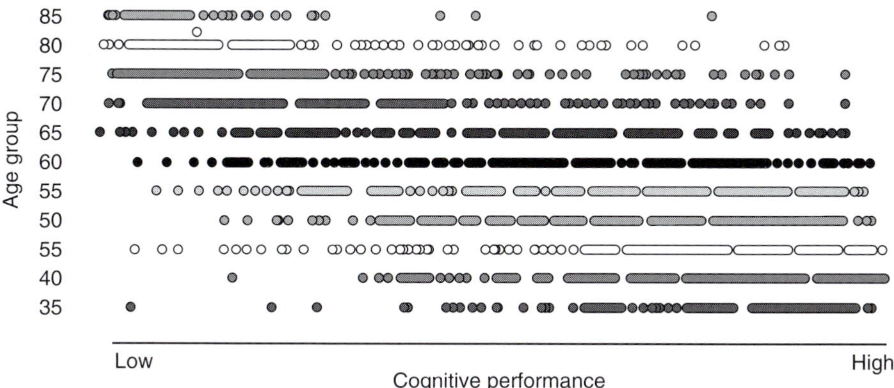

Figure 4.1 Distribution of average cognitive performance levels in persons between 35 and 85 years. *Source:* The figure is from Nyberg et al, 2012.[15] Data are based on two repeated measurements over five years in 1463 persons from a random population-based sample, the Swedish Betula study.[16]

levels of cognitive performance among aging persons. At higher ages, variability in cognitive performance between individuals typically increases.[15,16] As illustrated in Figure 4.1, this means that at age 70 or 80, many individuals still outperform a typical person at 40 or 45 years of age.

To determine if a certain level of cognitive performance is the result of an underlying neuropathological condition or not, we need more evidence than performance at a specific occasion. The term "cognitive decline" is often used to describe a lower-than-expected cognitive performance at a certain age, both in clinical and research settings, even when it is only based on the performance on a specific occasion, or during a very limited period. The term "decline" obviously denotes a change of performance, not a level of performance, and cannot logically be established except through repeated measurements over time. Failure to do so, may introduce two types of errors: assuming that an unusual low level of performance reflects cognitive decline, although this level is actually typical for this individual, and second, to miss that a relatively high level of performance could represent a pronounced decline, with a probable underlying neuropathology, from an even higher level that was previously typical for this individual. These errors are illustrated in Figure 4.2, where person C represents the first kind of misclassification, and the second error is for person A, exemplified by the introductory case, Emma – if we only base our evaluation on the cognitive performance at time point 2. The wide spread use of the term "cognitive decline," based on performance at a single occasion, has consequently been criticized.[17–19]

Although mild cognitive impairment (MCI) was originally proposed as a transition phase between normal cognitive functioning and AD, the originally proposed criteria did not include establishment of cognitive decline in the true sense (through repeated measurements).[13] Consequently, many patients who fulfilled these criteria did not progress to AD or any other form of dementia, and some of them even reverted to normal cognitive functioning.[14,20] In clinical and research settings, follow-up of the patient with sensitive neuropsychological tests and getting detailed medical history from patient and caregiver is therefore central. The importance of assessment over time to establish a MCI diagnosis was reflected in the revised MCI criteria from 2004.[21]

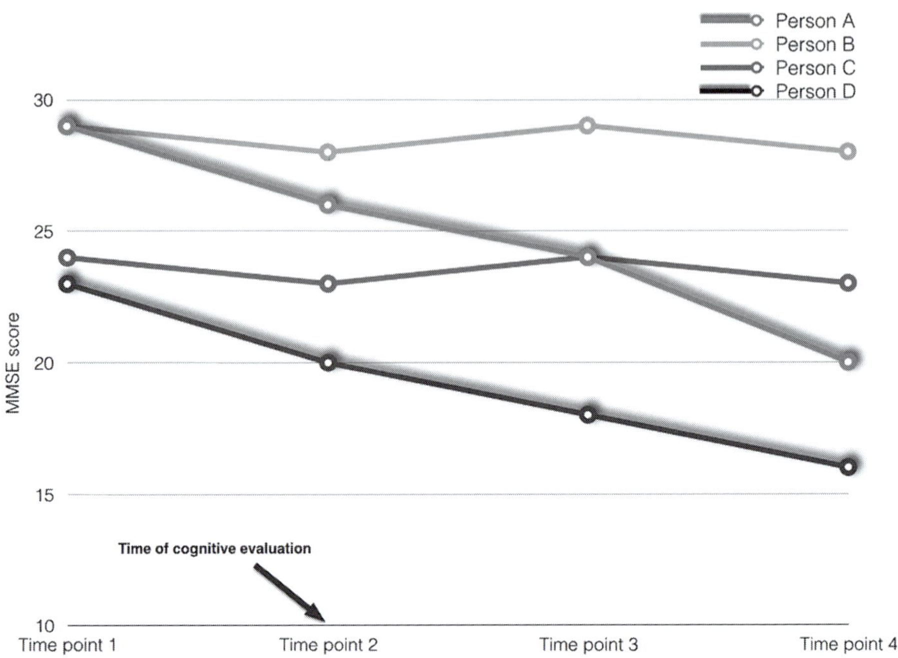

Figure 4.2 Illustration of four hypothetical cognitive change trajectories.

Brain Reserve and True Cognitive Decline

Brain reserve is a concept that is often used to account for differences in cognitive performance within a specific age cohort, due to differences in exposures with long-term effects on brain function.[22] Already decades ago, some classical experiments demonstrated that an enriched environment can increase cortical thickness and total brain weight in rodents.[23] Enriched animals also showed a richer neuronal dendritic network and improved learning abilities compared to less stimulated animals.[24] A large number of epidemiological studies on humans have shown that education especially,[25,26] but probably also other forms of intellectual stimulation during the whole life-course, is associated with lower dementia risk.[27] The core of the brain reserve hypothesis is that a brain with rich neural networks, at least partly as a result of prior stimulation, has better ability to resist and compensate against an underlying neurodegenerative disease process.[28] Empirical data support a number of factors that seem to help building such a brain reserve, including education, a range of other intellectual activities, physical exercise, and social factors.[29] Related to the brain reserve hypothesis is also the finding of a probable link between a higher cognitive capacity / intelligence early in life and a lower risk of dementia in old age.[30]

The brain reserve hypothesis builds closely on previously well-established characteristics of the nervous system, such as its plasticity; it has long been known that the brain is capable of repairing itself and of reallocating neural processes after injury to regions adjacent to the injured one and that this ability is more pronounced in younger individuals. As mentioned above, the effects of enriched environments on neural networks, dendritic spines, and synapses, which are all related to the brain's capacity to be modified by experience, are also well known. The concept of brain reserve can be viewed as a conceptual tool to explain individual differences in latency between the point of disease initiation and clinical diagnosis, although brain reserve probably has little to add to understanding why the disease process was initiated in the first place. The well-established association between higher education and lower dementia incidence, illustrates this point. More recent findings have shown that education is often associated with higher cognitive performance, but not with less cognitive decline.[31,32] This should mean that persons with high education typically have a longer period of cognitive decline before their cognition has dropped to a level where criteria are met for a dementia diagnosis, and when it does, that the disease at the neuropathological level has reached a more advanced stage,[33] as exemplified in the initial case description of Emma. This may also be the reason why a highly educated person often has a faster clinical progression of the disease after the time of an AD diagnosis.[31]

In summary, individual differences in brain reserve can complicate evaluations of cognitive health status and further highlight the need of follow-up examinations to detect true cognitive decline.

Persons with Dementia

Dementia, or major neurocognitive disorder in the recent DSM-V,[34] is an umbrella term for different conditions that contribute to severe impairment of cognition. Estimations say that around 47 million persons worldwide had a dementia diagnosis in 2015, a number projected to increase to 131 million in 2050.[35] The main reason behind this projection is an expected continued global increase in life expectancies, especially in low- and middle-income countries. The importance of age as a major driving force behind this development is illustrated by the fact that the proportion of persons with dementia approximately doubles with every 5 years of increased age after the age of 65; dementia prevalence is around 2–3 percent in populations between 65 and 70 years and grows to around 40 percent among persons above 85. Some recent studies have reported that prevalence or age-specific incidence rates within different age cohorts could be decreasing,[36–38] while other studies have failed to confirm such a trend in other populations.[39] In any case, these possible decreases do not nearly compensate for the added numbers produced by the growing proportion of an elderly population.

The most common dementia diagnosis is Alzheimer disease (AD), usually accounting for around 60–70 percent of dementia cases in different regions of the world, followed by vascular dementia (VaD) (15–30 percent of all cases) and Lewy-Body dementia (LBD) (5–15 percent).[40–44] Less common types of dementia include frontotemporal dementia (FTD), Parkinson dementia, and alcohol dementia. It is difficult to say whether reported variation in prevalences between regions and, e.g., between urban and rural areas, reflect differences in the quality of the studies, in diagnostic procedures, differential survival effects, or have other causes.[45] Although most reviews seems to conclude that the real variation is probably small across world regions, it has been recognized that both all-cause dementia and AD prevalence may be considerably lower among old people in parts of India[46] and sub-Saharan Africa,[47] for reasons yet unknown.

In reality, persons can suffer from more than one type of dementing disorders and brain pathology at the same time, and especially in old age it is common with vascular cognitive impairment along with other dementia types, probably making "mixed dementia" the most common condition, especially among the oldest old.[48] With this in mind, it may be more adequate to conceptualize dementia as a condition where vascular and neurodegenerative

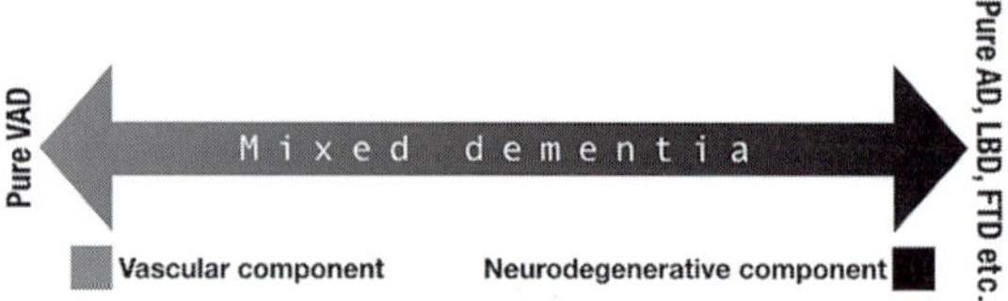

Figure 4.3 Continuous contribution of neurodegenerative and vascular components in dementia.

components combine and contribute to various degrees, rather than as distinct types, as illustrated in Figure 4.3.

We currently lack cure and disease-modifying treatments for neurodegenerative dementia types with still partly unknown and complex mechanisms such as AD and FTD. On the other hand, vascular and mixed cognitive impairment offers possibilities for several prevention and treatment interventions (see Chapter 1, 2, and 7–9).

Alzheimer's Disease

Alzheimer disease (AD) is the most common form of dementia, a progressive disease with an average survival time after diagnosis of around five years,[49–51] but with variation in survival time due to age at time of diagnosis, severity of the disease at the time of diagnosis and with a trend towards longer survival time for more recent diagnoses.[52] At present no pharmaceutical treatment has been found to cure or even halt its progress. A distinction is usually made between the familial (early onset) and sporadic (late-onset) AD. The rare familial type, with a prevalence of only around 1–2 percent typically affects a person already between 40 and 50 years of age, or even earlier. As the inheritance is autosomal dominant, children to a parent with this mutation will have a 50 percent chance of inheriting the allele, that can either be a mutation in the amyloid precursor protein (APP), presenilin-1 (PS1), or presenilin-2 (PS2) genes. The majority of AD cases have the sporadic form of the disease that is multifactorial and both environmental and genetic risk factors, and their interplay affects if and when a person develops the disease (see below).

The familial early onset form of AD resembles late-onset sporadic AD in many ways, but symptoms differ in some respects (e.g., in terms of motor functions), and biologically, familial AD may be associated with higher amyloid burden and a more aggressive progression of the disease.[53,54] Research on animal models with the aim of developing drugs against the common late-onset AD still seem to be based on the assumption that familial AD is basically the same disease as late onset AD; the common method in this type of research is to study pharmaceutical effects on animals with genetic mutations of the same kind as found in familial AD. Drugs that have successfully relieved animals from their amyloid burdens, building on the dominant amyloid cascade hypothesis as a crucial and causal process in AD development,[55] have not yet relieved humans with the common sporadic type of AD from their symptoms – or been able to halt the progression of the disease.[51] Earlier initiation of the treatment might change this situation, building on the assumption that the amyloid mechanisms addressed by a majority of drug trials are still valid, an assumption that remains to be verified in the face of recent doubts.[56–58] New proposed criteria to detect prodromal AD, relying on biomarkers to a higher extent than before,[59] should at least enable the diagnoses to be established earlier in the disease process, and thus to test this hypothesis.

Other processes seen in AD development, such as synaptic and mitochondrial dysfunction, inflammation, and oxidative stress,[60] have so far also not served as a basis for successful pharmaceutical strategies. Overall, during the last 30 years, over 200 experimental drugs to cure or halt AD have failed.[61]

Clinical Procedures to Establish Cognitive Impairment and Dementia

When a person comes to a medical clinic to examine their memory, they often do so because they, or their relatives, are worried that the patient has a cognitive impairment that indicates early dementia. Problems to perform cognitive tasks may, however, result from a number of other causes, such as depression, severe stress, sleep problems, age-related decline – or that a low level of cognitive performance is typical and normal for the particular patient. As dementia is usually a severely disabling condition with a prevalence of around 40 percent in persons over 85, it is easy to understand why many elderly persons fear to become victims. A natural consequence is an elevated sensitivity to symptoms that may indicate dementia, such as memory problems, symptoms that previously in life may not have been a source of worry. The doctor is thus presented with the task to determine what is behind the worries presented; do objective indications of early dementia exist?

There are several considerations that need to be made and combined in order to perform this task in a reliable way. One is to investigate evidence of an existing progress of symptoms. As we emphasize throughout this chapter, most types of dementia are characterized by a prolonged cognitive decline that eventually produces clinical symptoms that qualify for a dementia diagnosis. This is especially true for dementia types with a neuropathological origin, such as the common Alzheimer disease, but also for dementia types like fronto-temporal dementia (FTD) and Lewy-Body dementia (LBD). In the recent DSM-V criteria, establishing a preceding cognitive decline is stated as a prerequisite to determine that a person has dementia,[34] which means that cognitive decline, as opposed to poor cognitive performance, has been given a higher status compared to previous DSM versions. If this is a returning patient and previous cognitive testing has been performed, the existence of this criterion can be determined in an objective and reliable manner through repeated testing and comparisons with previous performance. The first step should therefore be to investigate if cognitive performance data can be accessed, either from the same clinic or from elsewhere.

Without prior cognitive measurements to compare with, we are left with the information that can be collected from patients and relatives when the clinical evaluation starts. We should, however, be aware that we will not be able to evaluate cognitive decline, and thereby the probability of an underlying dementia disease, based on cognitive performance at only one point in time, as previously justified (see Figure 4.2). A better option at this stage is to obtain other types of data that could indicate progression. This can be done in a way that is easier and more reliable than might be assumed – by asking the patient and preferably also close informants. The validity of such questions was illustrated in a study by Rönnlund et al in 2015 on 2034 elderly dementia-free persons in Sweden, as part of the Betula project.[62] They showed that especially one of the three questions – "Does anyone close to you (family, friends) think that you have a poor memory?" – clearly outperformed an extensive cognitive test battery as a predictor of future dementia. The other two questions, that were also superior to baseline cognitive testing, were related to a self-evaluation of cognitive ability in comparison with others of the same age and to how they perceived their memory today compared to five years ago.

To exemplify, persons who said that close persons often, or usually, complained about their memory, were over 4 times as likely to have a dementia diagnosis within 10 years, compared to persons who were unaware of such complaints. Of special interest in this context is that the adjustment for cognitive performance at baseline did not affect the power of this prediction. One interpretation of these results is that when close persons complain about memory problems in someone they know very well, they do that because they have noticed a deterioration, i.e., that this remark is an indicator of cognitive decline. Other studies on subjective cognitive decline as a predictor of subsequent dementia point in the same direction; that the person's own observation of cognitive deterioration could be a decent substitute when more objective evidence from repeated cognitive testing is lacking.[63] The Informant Questionnaire on Cognitive Decline in the Elderly (IQCODE) is one of the most commonly used and has been found highly reliable with a Cronbachs alfa of >0.90, at least as efficient in predicting future decline as standard cognitive testing, even compared to repeated cognitive testing.[64] Several reviews report sensitivity and specificity to predict future dementia of similar ranges (up to 0.8–0.9) as the combined use of $A\beta 1$–42 and T-tau/P-tau in CSF (see below).[65,66] The test has also been reported to perform very well in nonwestern settings.[67] It should, however, be noted that the samples in different studies have been heterogeneous, that many studies have been deemed to suffer from potential biases, and that the types of informants and study settings may affect the predictive efficiency of the instrument.[66] In conclusion, informants are a valuable source of information to evaluate if cognitive decline has preceded the visit to the physician, in combination with cognitive testing and especially in the absence of prior cognitive testing.

In the clinical examination of the patient, it should be observed that episodic memory is not the only cognitive domain that could be affected by an underlying dementia disease, not even in very early stages of AD. It is therefore important to make a broad evaluation of cognitive decline in different cognitive domains, including executive functions and functions related to daily living. To determine whether subjective cognitive complaints reflect an underlying dementia is a complex process where more information from more sources is always an advantage. This also includes information from relatives and other persons who are close to the patient. To exemplify, in a study on over 4000 persons without cognitive impairment at baseline, agreement between patients and informants on the existence of cognitive problems was associated with a fourfold incidence of subsequent cognitive impairment, a conversion rate twice as high as when only the participant or the informant reported a cognitive problem at baseline.[68]

The emphasis of decline means that this part of the evaluation should focus on gradual changes within the last few years, rather than a stable, but unsatisfactory cognitive function – or the opposite; a sudden drop in function. Both of these deviations from a gradual decline suggest that the subjective problems could have other causes than an underlying progressive neuropathology. As mentioned, there are many other possible reasons for both subjective complaints and poor cognitive performance in testing. Although cognitive decline, rather than a low level of performance, is considered as a prerequisite for a dementia diagnosis, even cognitive decline could have other reasons, such as incidence of depression, accumulating cerebrovascular events, or other conditions that have developed over time. To exclude such causes during the clinical examination, neuropsychiatric and neuropsychological testing is an essential part of the diagnostic procedure at this stage.

The use of biomarkers is becoming more common also in clinical practice to obtain a more reliable evaluation when cognitive problems with an underlying brain pathology cannot be excluded. Some form of neuroimaging, at present mainly the use of MRI, is nowadays standard procedure to examine if structural brain abnormalities can support a diagnosis of possible cognitive impairment. Positron emission tomography (PET) is not only used in research to trace different molecules of interest in the brain, but sometimes also in complicated clinical cases. Levels of protein molecules in CSF (at present mainly amyloids and tau) can also be used to support a diagnosis of possible early Alzheimer disease. Much of this rapid development, and related suggestions for new diagnostic procedures, has a focus on early diagnosis of Alzheimer disease and even to differentiate different AD subtypes.[69] There is at present no consensus on how these procedures should be performed, including how to differentiate between different types of dementia, and the recent DSM-V manual also does not prescribe them. To exemplify, a recent meta-analysis concluded that a combination of decreased levels of $A\beta 1\text{–}42$ and elevated levels of T-tau or P-tau in cerebrospinal fluid can distinguish early cases of AD from persons without the disease with sensitivity and a specificity of up to 90 percent.[70] This may seem impressive, but it still means that at least one out of ten persons with an underlying AD is unrecognized and also that one out of ten persons without the disease will be falsely diagnosed – if a diagnosis should solely rely on these measures. It should also be noted that this reported predictive power is at least not dramatically higher than the one reported for informant interviews (see above). When it comes to predicting conversion from MCI to AD, the combined efficiency of $A\beta$ and T-tau/P-tau is still rather limited.[70] It therefore seems likely that future recommendations will include several biomarkers, including both brain imaging and CSF markers, and that in addition specific patterns of convergence between them will be identified to discriminate between different pathological types and subtypes. It is beyond the scope of this chapter to give a detailed account of the rapid development in this field. It is also not a very bold prediction that the methods we use today will soon be outdated and replaced by more sophisticated ones, both in the case of neuroimaging, CSF markers and possibly also other techniques to better reflect normal and abnormal brain functioning.

In Figure 4.4, we summarize the different steps we have described above with special relevance for a person without a prior diagnosis of any cognitive impairment. This figure is supplemented by Table 4.1 for more detailed description and comments on each of the diagnostic phases in Figure 4.4.

The procedure we have outlined will have to be adapted to different circumstances and settings, e.g., if the patient has been referred from another clinic and some of the examinations that we suggest have already been performed – or if the patient already has a dementia diagnosis that needs to be validated. Different clinics will in addition have different resources and skills to perform other types of testing than the ones we have outlined. We would also like to emphasize that the proposed procedure builds on common present recommendations, on clinical experience, and on recent clinical research. We can expect that new knowledge will lead to more sensitive diagnostic tools, revised diagnostic criteria, and hopefully also to more efficient therapeutic methods. On the other hand, even if technology should change the way we collect some of these types of data, we think that the combined evidence from several sources – from the patient and informants and from cognitive testing and biomarkers, with an emphasis on establishing cognitive decline rather than level of performance – will guide clinical decisions for many years to come.

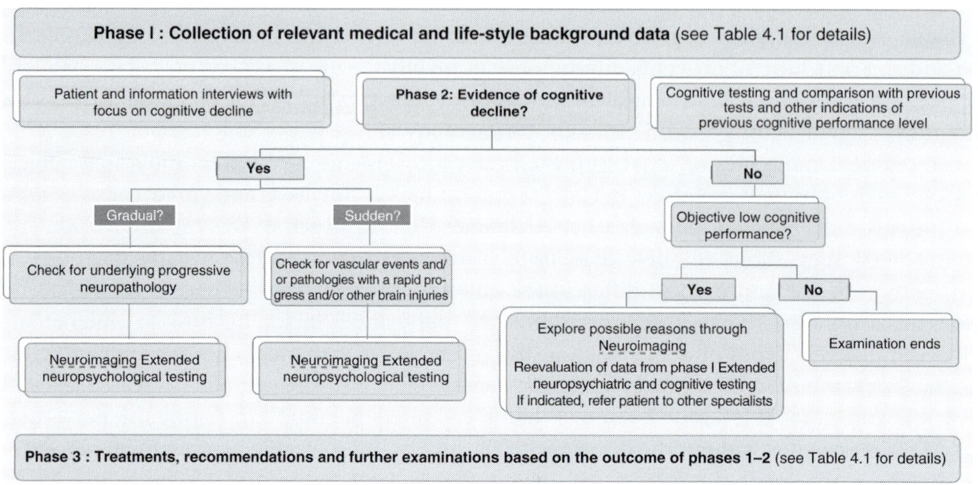

Figure 4.4 Suggested diagnostic procedure for a patient with cognitive complaints, but without prior diagnosis of cognitive impairment.

Nonpharmacological Strategies to Prevent or Postpone Dementia

The failure to find effective pharmaceutical treatment against AD and other types of dementia raises the question if there could be other options. A great number of epidemiological studies have revealed associations between a number of vascular, lifestyle and psychosocial factors that possibly could be translated into nonpharmacological strategies to prevent or postpone dementia. Among factors with a "protective" association against dementia are physical exercise,[71] a generally active lifestyle,[72] social interactions,[73] and a "Mediterranean" diet (including regular consumption of olive oil, fish, fruit, and vegetables),[72] that has also been found to counteract cognitive decline.[74] Proposed risk factors include midlife hypertension and hypercholesterolemia,[75] diabetes,[76] midlife obesity,[77,78] smoking, loneliness,[79,80] depression,[81] hopelessness,[82,83] and stress.[84,85] In the context of this book, it is interesting to observe that several of these factors, with an obvious relation to the risk of vascular cognitive impairment, also increase the risk of Alzheimer disease, such as hypertension[75] and diabetes[86] in midlife. It remains to demonstrate the mechanisms behind these associations, e.g., whether they actually contribute to eliciting AD and through which pathways, or whether they simply add to the cognitive impairment and thereby to an earlier assessment and detection of AD. However, from a pragmatic point of view these associations still represent a group of modifiable factors with a potential to decrease the risk of cognitive impairment. The reported decline in dementia prevalence in some Western countries[51] has been linked to these factors, e.g., better treatment of BP, reduced incidence of stroke, lower frequency of smoking and higher education.[37]

Interactions between Genetic and Environmental Factors

Another observation from several observational association studies is that the most important genetic factor, the *ApoE 4* allele, in itself, when other factors are adjusted for, implies approxi-mately a two- to three-fold risk increase of AD, comparable in magnitude with several lifestyle

Table 4.1 Details of procedures and considerations in the proposed diagnostic procedure for persons without a previous diagnosis of cognitive impairment (Figure 4.4)

Phase 1: Collection of relevant medical and lifestyle background information

- Vascular/metabolic and lifestyle risk factors, including dementia risk score
- Medical history, including previous stroke, cardiovascular disease, hypertension, cancer
- Recent major life events of psychosocial significance
- History of falls
- Family history
- Cognitive and functional tests, including MMSE and gait
- Screening for depression, sleep problems, stress and burnout, and trauma
- Psychosocial status, including cohabitant status, social integration, and feelings of loneliness
- Current medication list and history of medication
- Basic lab tests to exclude somatic disorders or conditions, including vitamin B12, thyroidea, cholesterol, and relevant inflammation markers
- Blood pressure and BMI

Phase 2: Evaluation of cognitive decline over time

- Anamnesis from patient and from informant, through interview and validated questionnaires
- If possible, access results from previous cognitive testing and compare with current cognitive status
- Proxy indications of previous mental capacity: education, school grades, and professional activities
- See Figure 4.4 for the different diagnostic strategies, depending on the three possible outcomes:

    a)　no evidence of cognitive decline
    b)　gradual decline (at least observable for more than 9–12 months)
    c)　decline that is more sudden.

    Neuroimaging needed for diagnostic purposes for patients in category b) and c)

Phase 3: Treatments, recommendations, and further examinations based on the outcome of phases 1–2

1. All patients are given health advice and treatment according to the most probable cause of their cognitive concerns, in line with best available knowledge and recommendations at the time. All patients, including the ones without indications of cognitive decline or impairment, are also given both general and tailored lifestyle and health recommendations to decrease the risk of, or to counteract, cognitive impairment. This means that all patients will get advice and support in the following areas:

    - Management of vascular and metabolic risk factors
    - Dietary counseling (including medical food)
    - Advice on physical exercise
    - Cognitively stimulating activities and/or cognitive training programs

2. Persons who possibly have other causes (not related to a neuropathology or vascular disease) for a diagnostically confirmed cognitive impairment are either treated for these other conditions or referred to specialist care. (Obviously this also applies to any other medical condition that was detected.) Examples of cognitive relevance could be post-traumatic stress syndrome (PTSD), depression, a suspected brain tumor, or insomnia.
3. For persons with a probable or possible dementia as underlying cause, the best available treatment for the specific type of dementia at the time is given.

Table 4.1 (cont.)

> a. It is important to determine the type(s) of underlying neuropathology, and if uncertain, to reinforce the importance of healthy lifestyle changes to counteract further cognitive decline. In contrast to medication of neuropathological dementia types, there will be no side effects from these measures (see later sections of this chapter).
> b. Most patients with early cognitive symptoms from an underlying neuropathology will need follow-up and further examinations to establish the type of neuropathology that is the major cause of their symptoms.
>
> 4. Patients with a diagnosis of suspected or confirmed cognitive impairment are scheduled for revisit. Patients without cognitive decline, or signs of cognitive impairment, are invited to contact the clinic again if they find reasons of concern in the future.

factors. Several studies indicate however that the contribution of this genetic factor to AD increases significantly when it is combined with potentially modifiable risk factors such as physical inactivity, alcohol and smoking,[87] and with depressive feelings[82,83] and living alone.[88]

Apolipoprotein E (ApoE) is a lipoprotein that can be produced in the liver and in the brain by astrocytes. It has several biological roles, including cholesterol transport to the liver and in the nervous system, and transport of fatty acids and phospholipids. The prevalence of the three isoforms ApoE2, ApoE3 and ApoE4 varies somewhat across populations, and this is especially true for *ApoE4*.[89] In the Nordic countries the prevalence of *ApoE4* is typically around 25–30 percent,[89] while the prevalence in the Caucasian population at large has been estimated to around 15 percent.[90] The *ApoE4* allele is not only associated with a higher risk for AD but also for cardiovascular disease and a poorer prognosis after traumatic brain injury.[91] One meta-analysis estimated the average odds ratio for AD to 2.7 (CI 2.2.–3.2) for *ApoE3/4* carriers versus non-*ApoE4* carriers (ApoE3/3 carriers) in the Caucasian population, and up to 14.9 (CI 10.8–20.6) for *ApoE4/4* in the same population.[90]

The mechanisms behind the risk increase for AD as a function of *ApoE4* status is still partly unknown, but several studies have reported that *ApoE4* is also associated with higher amyloid burden and neurofibrillary tangles.[92] The possibility of an indirect link is indicated by the fact that *ApoE4* is also associated with other risk factors for dementia such as depression[93] and cardiovascular disease.[94]

Going from Observation to Intervention: Some Critical Issues

The critical question is to what degree associations from previous epidemiological studies can be translated into interventions to effectively counteract cognitive decline and dementia. The realism of this translation rests on the assumption that candidate factors derived from these associations reflect a causative role in the development of, or protection against, cognitive impairment. There are several reasons why this assumption may not be valid. The most obvious reason relates to the inherent methodological weakness in observational association studies, compared to a randomized experimental design. When adherence to a certain lifestyle pattern, such as being physically active, living in a cohabitant relationship, or embarking on a long education, is self-selected, these choices are also associated with other factors. The classical method to consider potential confounders in observational association studies is to statistically adjust for them in an attempt to isolate the association with the factor of interest. But as it is not possible to adjust for all possible confounders, residual associations can never be fully excluded. Examples of factors that are rarely adjusted for in epidemiological association studies are childhood experiences, personality, and other genetic factors than the *ApoE4*. The possibility that largely unknown genetic factors contribute to the development of AD is indicated by twin studies where concordance rates suggest that the total heritability of AD could be over 50 percent,[95] i.e., far higher than the contribution from the *ApoE4* allele. Another reason for skepticism is the fact that genes interplay with environmental factors, exemplified by the fast-growing field of epigenetics. This could mean that the attempt to separate the contribution of genetic factors from lifestyle factors and other environmental exposures is basically misleading.

A second complication in the interpretation of observational association studies is the possibility of reverse causation. Alzheimer disease in particular develops over the course of many years or even decades before it can be diagnosed, which means that "dementia-free" persons at baseline may still have AD in the preclinical stage of the disease, a condition that potentially could have an effect on the variable of interest, e.g., on how socially or physically active a person is. The neurodegenerative process and disease-related behavioral changes may also affect biological factors like weight and blood pressure, which often decline several years before the diagnosis and may lead to the observation that low body mass index and blood pressure are often related with dementia in shorter-term and cross-sectional studies.[96] Thus, an association between such factors and a subsequent dementia could potentially reflect reverse causation. Only longitudinal studies with an extensive follow-up time can hope to avoid the risk of reverse causation, but as the typical length of subclinical disease development is uncertain, it is difficult to determine how long the follow-up period needs to be. If it can be assumed that prodromal preclinical cognitive decline is a conservative estimate of the initiation of the subclinical disease process, such decline has been reported up to 12 years before diagnosis,[97] although other studies have found this period to be considerably shorter.[98] Especially if we assume that cognitive decline is the result of a neuropathological process that has already progressed in order to manifest as measurable decline in cognition,[99] it is probably a conservative estimate that the follow-up time needs to be at least 15 years to avoid the risk of reverse causation. This is a requirement that few prospective epidemiological association studies have met.

A third reason for skepticism against the idea of translating between association and intervention studies relates to time; in order to establish a causal effect on dementia risk, a minimal requirement for an association study is a very long follow-up period. Several of the best association studies show associations between lifestyle factors already in midlife and the risk of cognitive impairment in old age, as illustrated in Figure 4.5. The question then arises: will interventions based on such factors be effective to prevent or delay cognitive impairment in old age and/or in persons who already show some cognitive impairment – or who already have dementia?

As a consequence of these and other methodological issues, a NIH expert panel concluded in 2010, after a quality-based selection of 275 studies out of over 6000 in total, that quality of evidence was too low to permit any safe conclusions concerning factors that could either increase or decrease the risk of cognitive decline, for neither pharmacological nor nonpharmacological approaches, but with one exception: this panel found cognitive training to have a well-documented, albeit small effect on cognitive performance.[100] The main reason for exception of cognitive training was the existence of a randomized control intervention study of high quality, the ACTIVE study,[101] that confirmed results from previous association studies.[100] The ACTIVE study included 2832 healthy elderly persons who were randomly distributed into four equal

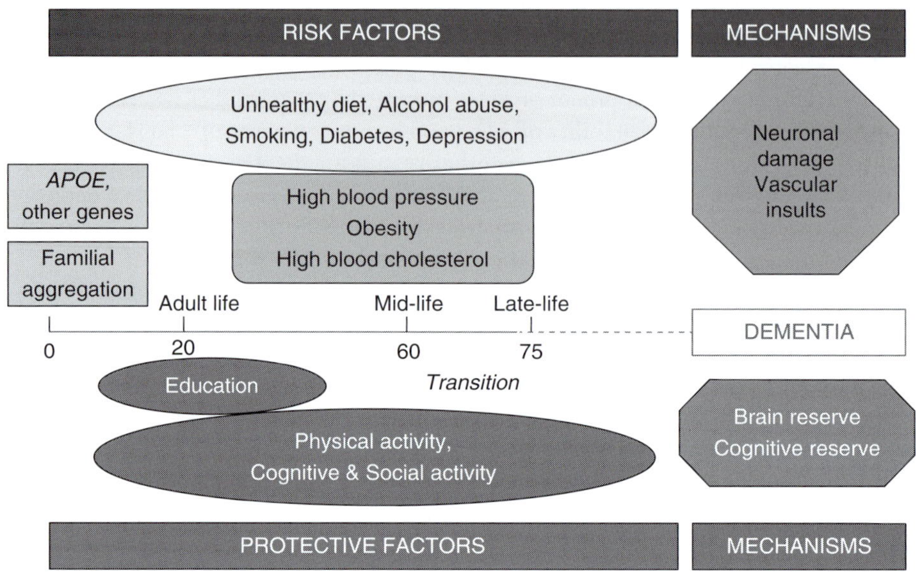

Figure 4.5 Dementia and cognitive impairment: importance of life-long exposure to multiple factors.

groups who did memory training, reasoning training, executive speed training, or served as a passive control.[101] The intervention groups performed 10 training sessions during the first year and in addition a subsample of participants (around 45 percent) performed 8 booster sessions during the following 2 years. The effects on cognition and daily living were evaluated 10 years after the initiation of the study for all participants. In summary, the results indicated remaining effects after 10 years for both reasoning and processing speed training, but no effects from memory training, and these effects only pertained to the cognitive domain that had been trained (no transfer effects to other domains). The effect size was larger for processing speed training (effect size = 0.66, 99 percent CI = 0.43–0.88) than for reasoning training (effect size 0.23, 99 percent CI = 0.09–0.38).[101] At the time of the NIH evaluation, this well-designed study was regarded as a convincing demonstration of a real long-term impact of a unimodal intervention on cognitive performance in old persons without cognitive impairment at baseline.

From Unimodal to Multimodal Interventions

After the publication of the NIH expert panel review in 2010,[100] several randomized trials (RCT) have been performed in order to validate the findings from observational studies, especially for cognitive and physical activity. A recent meta-analysis of 17 original RCTSs concluded that computerized cognitive training in persons with mild cognitive impairment had a positive, but relatively modest effect (g=0.35 99 percent CI=0.20–0.51), whereas for persons with dementia, the effect was at best negligible.[102] This meta-analysis also reported that most of the individual studies were unable to demonstrate a significant effect and concluded that several of them suffered from a poor methodological design and insufficient statistical power.[102]

A similar picture appears to exist for physical exercise where no or small effects have been found on cognition in persons with mild cognitive impairment.[103] In persons with dementia, and in contrast with reported effects of cognitive training, a recent meta-analysis on 17 individual RCT studies concluded that aerobic physical exercise can be efficient to counteract further cognitive decline, independent of dementia type.[104]

For other factors, previously identified by association studies as potential intervention candidates, results have been even more disappointing. These include pharmacological studies on hormone replacement therapy (HRT), and nonsteroidal anti-inflammatory drugs (NSAIDs), both without positive effects on cognition. According to a recent review by Winblad et al,[51] the only single-drug approach that so far has showed some positive effects is for antihypertension medication, a conclusion that is in contrast with the even more pessimistic conclusion by the NIH expert panel review from 2010.[100]

In summary, when factors from observational studies with promising "protective" associations have been tested in randomized control trials, they have in general not lived up to the expectations. This indicates that the translation from association to intervention cannot always be done in a straightforward way. We have mentioned several possible reasons for this, including the incomplete handling of possible confounders in an association study, the risk of reverse causation, and the difference between an association over decades, started already in midlife, and an intervention during a relatively much shorter time period, starting later in older age. Another possibility relates to the interpretation of the results from previous observational association studies, where typically one factor at a time has been investigated, while adjusting for all other factors with available data that could modify the association between the "predictor" and the outcome of interest, usually cognitive impairment of some kind. If we consider the pattern of results from these studies, could this give clues to how an intervention could more realistically be designed to be effective?

One striking feature in the research body from association studies is the multitude of factors that seem to show associations with the risk of subsequent cognitive impairment (see Figure 4.5). It should also be evident from these factors that the association with cognitive impairment is not unique; the same factors are also related to a host of other health conditions, and this should apply both for factors with beneficial and adverse effects. A more holistic interpretation from this scenario is that they all contribute and combine to affect health in a nonspecific way, and that the specific disease outcome is determined by individual vulnerabilities, where genetic factors should have a special role. This line of reasoning, previously referred to as a "socio-genetic" disease model, in a previous study on social factors,[88] might have a wider relevance than for social factors, for any combination of factors that implies a burden on the biological system, thereby weakening biological resistance to disease development and making repair mechanisms more inefficient. This is illustrated in Figure 4.6.

The route from exposure to systemic burden to disease is probably not unidirectional. It seems highly likely that once a disease has developed, it will in itself constitute a burden that will weaken the system and increase the risk of further diseases. This is illustrated in Figure 4.6 by the thin arrows pointing back from the different possible diseases to the non-specific factor.

To exemplify in some more detail, in Figure 4.7 we have entered four lifestyle factors that could be of relevance both for the risk of cognitive impairment and for several other health conditions; immunological efficiency is suggested as a candidate systemic factor of relevance, and *ApoE4* is exemplified as a genetic factor that could make AD a relatively more probable ill health outcome. This model does not preclude the possibility that some factors, in addition to their systemic impacts, could imply a specific disease risk due to the nature of the exposure. In Figure 4.7 we have exemplified this with the specific risk increase of lung cancer from cigarette smoking.

We also propose that the different exposures should be regarded as interrelated (not illustrated in the figures). This assumption means that the presence of one exposure factor

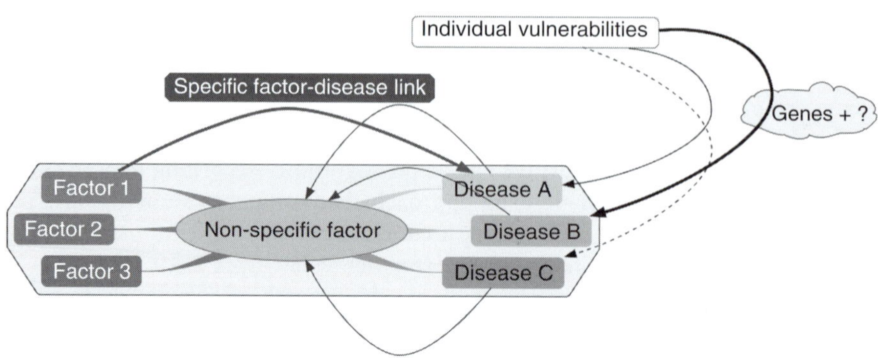

Figure 4.6 A systemic factor disease model to account for general and specific health effects from a multitude of exposures.

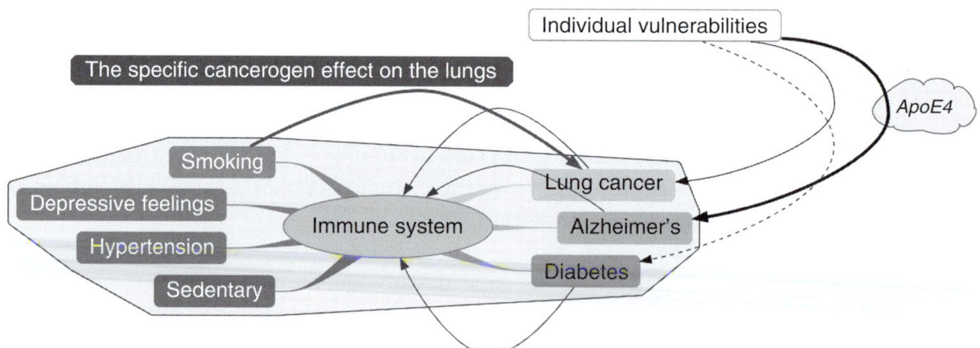

Figure 4.7 The systemic disease model exemplified.

often affects the probability of others also being present. To exemplify, sedentary behavior may both be affected by, and affect, the probability of hypertension, obesity, and smoking. Smoking may in a similar way affect the probability that a person is depressed, sedentary, and overweight – and the presence of at least some of these may in turn affect the risk of smoking. If exposures in this way are inter-related and dynamically affect each other, a strategy where these factors are investigated in isolation, e.g., through statistical adjustments, may be very different from how they function in real life and, when implemented unimodally in lifestyle interventions, may reduce their potential benefits.

We also need to recognize that specific genetic vulnerabilities do not simply affect the more probable disease outcome that results from general immunological inefficiency and dysfunction. Genes also affect both immunological function and the lifestyle choices people make. Many of the non-*APOE4* genes that have been recently discovered to either increase or decrease the risk of AD are related to immunological function.[105] Further research will have to verify if this, in line with the proposed model, means that some genes of relevance for immunological function also show common associations with several different diseases.

When applied to cognitive impairment and the possibility to prevent it, this line of thinking suggests that the common one-factor approach may be inadequate. A possible interpretation of the multitude of factors that show a long-term association with either increased or reduced risk of cognitive impairment is thus that they have combined and synergistic effects and that effective prevention should be based on such a multifactor approach. It also implies that research in this field could benefit from keeping an eye also on other diseases, rather than isolating the outcome to cognitive decline or impairment. In order to test the assumption that combined measures can be more efficient, several RCT studies have used both physical and cognitive training and compared the combined effect on cognition with the effect of training only one of them. A recent meta-analysis reviewed 20 such studies with a total of 2667 participants without cognitive impairment at baseline and found an effect size of 0.29 (p=0.001) for the combined intervention effect of physical and cognitive training. Although this effect was higher than for any of the unimodal interventions, the combined advantage was not significantly higher than for cognitive training alone.[106]

To take the hypothesis of a combined advantage one step further, three large randomized control studies, including a total of almost 6500 persons, combined several factors into multimodal interventions. One of these found an effect in the primary outcome of the study,[107] whereas the other two studies did not, although they reported interesting results from subgroup analyses.[108,109] In the following, we will take a closer look at each of them and compare outcomes, interventions, and the selection of participants as possible explanations for the difference in results and to suggest future developments.

The FINGER Study

The Finnish Geriatric Intervention Study (FINGER)[110] included 1260 participants, recruited from previous surveys in the general population of Finland. Inclusion criteria were dementia-free persons aged between 60 and 77 who had a CAIDE dementia risk score of at least 6 and who did not perform higher than average in cognitive tests. The purpose of these selection criteria were to estimate the effects in a population at higher dementia risk than the average elderly population. The participants were randomly assigned to a control group or a multimodal intervention group. Participants were not actively told into which group they were randomized, and research staff conducting outcome assessment were blinded. FINGER used an active control group where participants received health advice and they also met six times during the study period with either a nurse or a physician to monitor their cardiovascular health and to get medical advice. The multidomain intervention group had additional health checks and also participated in a program that combined physical and cognitive training, and nutritional guidance. During the first six months, a physiotherapist led the physical exercise sessions (aerobic, strength, and postural balance), and the participants were recommended to perform these exercises with increased intensity and frequency during the two years (three to five gym sessions per week during the second year). They had seven group sessions with nutritional advice and in addition three individual sessions with a nutritionist during the two years. Cognitive training was performed through a computerized program 2–3 times per week, introduced and reinforced through 10 group sessions during the intervention period. The difference between the active control and the intervention group is illustrated in Figure 4.8.

The main outcome in the FINGER study was change in cognitive performance, as measured by a Neuropsychological Test Battery (NTB), calculated both for global cognition and in addition for three different cognitive domains. Both the active control and the intervention group improved their overall cognitive performance, but the intervention group did so significantly more than the active control (25 percent higher improvement,

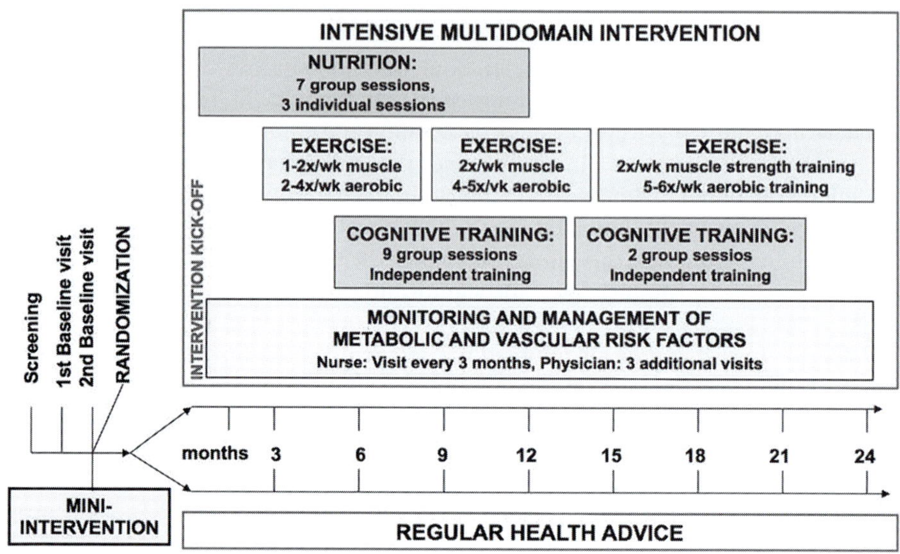

Figure 4.8 The active control group and the intervention group in the FINGER study. From Kivipelto et al (ref 110)

p=0.03).[107] Among separate cognitive domains (prespecified outcomes), the difference was especially large for executive functioning (83 percent difference) and processing speed (150 percent higher). There was also a significant intervention group advantage for complex memory (40 percent higher improvement in the intervention group). Further, the control group had 30 percent higher risk for cognitive decline. Positive results were also detected on several secondary outcomes (e.g., lifestyle factors, health-related quality of life).[107] The pattern of results for the three cognitive domains with a significant difference is illustrated in Figure 4.9.

Drop-out rate was only 12 percent during the two years, and drop-out rate was similar in both groups.[107] The study did not have any safety concerns.

The preDIVA study

The preDIVA study evaluated a multidomain intervention during 6 years where a total of 3526 participants were recruited through 26 health care centers with a total of 116 general practices in the Netherlands.[109] Of the 116 practices, 63 were randomly selected to implement the intervention protocol and the remaining 53 to serve as control with care as usual. The 1890 GP patients in the intervention group visited the clinic every four months during the six years that the intervention went on. During each visit, a nurse assessed their cardiovascular health and the exposure to various cardiovascular risk factors, including smoking, diet, physical activity, weight, and blood pressure. Tailored lifestyle advice was given to each participant based on these assessments, supplemented by motivational interviews. For participants with hypertension, diabetes, and/or dyslipidemia, adequate drug treatment was prescribed and optimized. The primary outcomes were incidence of dementia during the six years and level of disability development. The study found that both incidence of dementia (7 percent) and disability were the same between the intervention

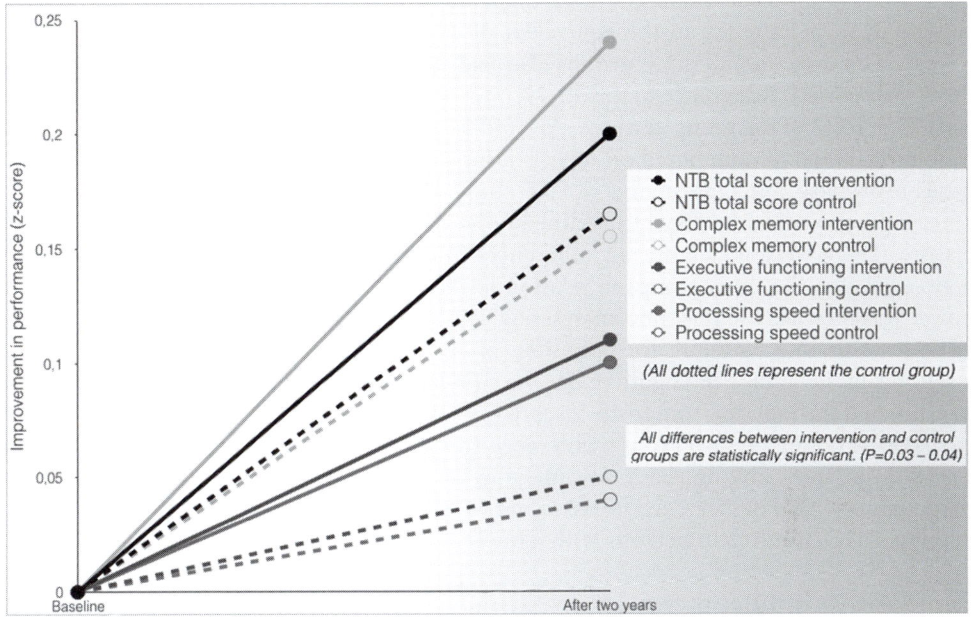

Figure 4.9 Effects of the FINGER intervention on global cognition and for three cognitive domains.

group and the control group.[109] One of the secondary outcomes in preDIVA was cognitive decline, but also for this outcome there was no difference between the two groups.[109] Subgroup analyses suggested a positive effect among persons with untreated hypertension at baseline.

The MAPT Study

The third large multimodal study to be discussed is the MAPT intervention study.[108] This study differs in relation to the other two by the inclusion of three intervention groups, in addition to a control group. The purpose of this design was to test if omega-3 polyunsaturated fatty acid supplementation or multidomain lifestyle intervention, alone or in combination, would prevent cognitive decline. The intervention went on for 3 years and included 1525 dementia-free patients from 13 memory clinics in France and Monaco who were randomized into 4 groups: 2 multidomain intervention groups with or without the omega-3 supplementation, a group with omega-3 supplementation alone, and a control group. Exclusion criteria were either dementia or a MMSE performance below a score of 24. To be included, the patients had to be over 70 years old and have at least one of the following: subjective memory complaints, slow gait speed, or limitation in at least one instrumental activity of daily living. The multidomain intervention consisted of 12 group sessions during the first two months and two reinforcement sessions at 12 and 24 months. These two-hour sessions included cognitive training and demonstration and advice of physical training that the participants were instructed to do at home, and nutritional guidance. For physical training, the participants were recommended to perform physical activity in their daily life to the equivalent of at least 30 min walking per day, five days a week. The three intervention groups also had three preventive consultations during the three-year period. Adherence to the intervention program was defined as participation in at least 75 percent of the group sessions. Around 54 percent of the participants adhered to the multimodal intervention based on this criterion.

The primary outcome in the MAPT study was cognitive decline, assessed through a neuropsychological battery at baseline and at follow-up, and calculated as a composite z score. There were no significant differences in cognitive decline during the three years between any of the three groups in relation to the placebo control group. When statistical power was increased in post hoc analyses by combining the two multidomain intervention groups (with and without the addition of omega-3), this combined group showed a significant advantage in cognitive decline in relation to the placebo control group, both as estimated through the composite z score (p=0.015) and through score change in MMSE (p=0.036). Pooling the two groups who received the omega-3 supplementation in the same way did not show any omega-3 advantage in relation to the control group. In addition, participants with a higher CAIDE risk score (6 or higher)[111] gained more from the multi-domain intervention than persons with a lower risk of dementia.[108]

Comparison between the Three Studies

Among the three multimodal interventions that have been described, the preDIVA study found no intervention effect at all, whereas the MAPT study found some effects, and the strongest effects were found in the FINGER study. Although all three studies used a multimodal intervention and shared many similar characteristics, in some important ways they were different. For example, the preDIVA included unselected participants from health care centers, the MAPT study used various recruitment methods including patient databases and advertisements, and FINGER used a population-based sample with an increased risk of dementia. The content and intensity of interventions was different between the studies: FINGER study was most intensive, with more visits and including active cognitive and exercise training in addition to advice. In the MAPT study, the multidomain sessions included cognitive training and advice for the other domains. In the preDIVA the intervention visits included lifestyle advice, and active treatment of vascular risk factors. The studies also differed in terms of primary outcomes (dementia versus cognitive change) and length (24–72 months). Some of these differences are presented in Table 4.2. Can these differences in study characteristics also explain the differences in results?

All three studies could be classified as a mixture of primary and secondary prevention, as the participants did not have clinical dementia at baseline, but, especially in MAPT, they may have had health problems that could indicate preclinical dementia, i.e., a neuropathological progress of the disease before clinical symptoms have started to emerge. In reality, this distinction between primary and secondary prevention is not as easy to make as it may seem, and it may also be more relevant for cognitive impairment with a neuropathological origin. When the origin is mainly vascular, it is less obvious to imagine a point when the subclinical disease process "starts," and thus when measures could be taken to avoid its initiation. In addition, even when cognitive impairment of a vascular origin has progressed, the aim could potentially be more ambitious than to attenuate symptoms and slow down further progress, as pointed out in other chapters of this book.

Table 4.2 Selected features that differ between the three multimodal studies

Features	preDiva	MAPT	Finger
Sample size	3526	1680	1260
Sample origin	Health care centers	patient databases, advertisements	Population-based
Age	70–78	>70	60–77
Inclusion criteria	dementia-free, no major health problems	dementia-free, subjective memory problems, slow gait, ADL limitations	dementia-free, but elevated risk of dementia
Length	72 months	36 months	24 months
Control	care as usual	placebo (pill)	regular health advice
Outcome	dementia incidence	cognitive change	cognitive change
Intervention	1) Nurse visits every 4 months with cardiovascular risk factor advice/ drug treatment	1) 43 multidomain group sessions with cognitive training, and advice on physical activity and nutrition and 3 individual preventive consultations. 2) Omega-3 polyunsaturated fatty acid supplementation 3) Multidomain + omega 3	1) Multidomain intervention with nutritional guidance (3 individual and 6 group visits); physical activity (resistance and balance training 2–3 times /week + advice for aerobic training); cognitive training (6 group sessions + independent computerized training); vascular risk management (6 nurse and doctor visits)

As the authors point out,[109] one reason why the preDIVA intervention did not show an effect could simply be that the actual difference in treatment between the two groups was not large enough; both groups were GP patients, and it can be assumed that also many of the patients in the control group received similar advice as in the intervention group; the intervention was built on Dutch GP-guidelines for cardiovascular risk management, i.e., guidelines that apply to all physicians in the Netherlands.[112] As this intervention specifically aimed to reduce dementia by improving cardiovascular health, it is of interest that the decrease by 2.1 and 1.2 units in systolic and diastolic blood pressure respectively, even though statistically significant with calculations based on around 3000 subjects, may not have been sufficient to make a difference in terms of dementia incidence. The mean systolic blood pressure was considerably reduced in both groups during the 6 years, but the mean systolic blood pressure levels at the end of study were still a high 148.0 in the intervention group and 149.6 in the control group. The choice of a dichotomous outcome (incidence of dementia versus not) in the preDIVA study could have further contributed to the absence of a visible effect, especially as the preDIVA participants were not selected based on baseline risk profile.

It is also of interest that the MAPT study found an effect specifically in participants with a CAIDE risk score above 6,[108] while a CAIDE risk score of 6 or more was an inclusion criterion in the FINGER study.[107]

The studies also differ somewhat in the choice of ingredients they included in the multimodal package. The MAPT study specifically tested the addition of omega-3 polyunsaturated fatty acids and found that they did not add to the multimodal intervention effect. Information of this type should have great value to guide development of future multimodal interventions. With only 1525 participants, this demonstration, however, came with a price; only when the 2 multimodal groups were combined (both with and without the addition of omega-3) did a significant effect emerge for the multimodal intervention.[108]

After the success with the multimodal approach in FINGER, this study has now become a model for several other intervention studies around the world, including in China, the US, Great Britain and Singapore. Harmonization of measures and designs between the different sites will enable data merging and more powerful subgroup analyses. Comparison between sites could also increase understanding of how the original FINGER design need to be adapted to consider important cultural differences between countries. The further development of the World Finger initiative can be followed through its dedicated website at http://wwfingers.com/

Future Directions

By careful comparison of contents, intensities, sample characteristics and other features in these and forthcoming multimodal intervention studies, complemented with post hoc calculations to test hypotheses that might emerge from these comparisons, it should be possible to identify types of multimodal interventions that will have the greatest benefit for different target groups. Even if such efforts can make future multimodal interventions much more efficient than the ones having been suggested and tested so far, it may, however, not be realistic that they can either cure all types of dementia, or prevent their corresponding neuropathological processes from being initiated in the first place. It is import to keep in mind that if such interventions are only moderately successful they could reduce the number of dementia cases by around 20 percent.[113] If they would be able to slow down the pathological process and postpone clinical dementia by an average of five years, this would produce a 50 percent decrease of the number of people with dementia in the world.[114]

Final Reflections

Much remains in order to establish optimal lifestyle patterns that can prevent and/or delay cognitive impairment in later life, but if lifestyle changes are made in line with the best available evidence, it is hard to imagine adverse side effects. The chances are also good that such changes may promote health in a more general way, rather than having a limited effect on only cognitive functioning and brain health. If the assumptions are correct behind the systemic health model we propose, it could be a good idea to change the overall lifestyle pattern, rather than adopting a unimodal approach, such as increasing physical exercise or switching to a particular diet, and to integrate these changes in daily life with other activities, rather than at special occasions. The things we do at one point in time affect other things we do at other times, and it may be the totality that matters in the end. Applied to research in the field, it may mean that future interventions should be even broader to include social, emotional, physical, vascular, sleep quality, artistic, and dietary factors, cleverly integrated rather than performed separately at special occasions.

References

1. Yang J, Wong A, Wang Z, et al. Risk factors for incident dementia after stroke and transient ischemic attack. *Alzheimers Dement.* 2015;**11**(1):16–23.

2. Finkel D, Reynolds CA, McArdle JJ, Pedersen NL. Cohort differences in trajectories of cognitive aging. *J Gerontol, Series B.* 2007;**62**(5): P286–P294.

3. Flynn JR. Massive IQ gains in 14 nations: what IQ tests really measure. *Psychol Bull.* 1987;**101**(2):171–191.

4. Fozard JL, Vercryssen M, Reynolds SL, Hancock PA, Quilter RE. Age differences and changes in reaction time: the Baltimore Longitudinal Study of Aging. *J Gerontol.* 1994;**49**(4):P179–P189.

5. Hultsch DF, MacDonald SWS, Dixon RA. Variability in reaction time performance of younger and older adults. *J Gerontol, Series B.* 2002;**57**(2):P101–P115.

6. Hultsch DF, MacDonald SW, Hunter MA, Levy-Bencheton J, Strauss E. Intraindividual variability in cognitive performance in older adults: comparison of adults with mild dementia, adults with arthritis, and healthy adults. *Neuropsychology.* 2000;**14** (4):588–598.

7. Dhaliwal G. Premature closure? Not so fast. *BMJ Qual Saf.* 2017;**26**(2):87–89.

8. Links S. Personality and psychopathology: the dangers of premature closure. *World Psychiatry.* 2011;**10**(2):109–110.

9. Garcia-Ptacek S, Eriksdotter M, Jelic V, Porta-Etessam J, Kareholt I, Palomo SM. Subjective cognitive impairment: towards early identification of Alzheimer disease. *Neurología (English Edition).* 2016;**31** (8):562–571.

10. Blazer D. Neurocognitive disorders in DSM-5. *Am J Psychiatry.* 2013;**170** (6):585–587.

11. Reisberg B, Gauthier S. Current evidence for subjective cognitive impairment (SCI) as the pre-mild cognitive impairment (MCI) stage of subsequently manifest Alzheimer's disease. *Int Psychogeriatr.* 2008;**20**(1):1–16.

12. Jonker C, Geerlings MI, Schmand B. Are memory complaints predictive for dementia? A review of clinical and population-based studies. *Int J Geriatr Psychiatry.* 2000;**15**(11):983–991.

13. Petersen RC, Roberts RO, Knopman DS, et al. Mild cognitive impairment: ten years later. *Arch Neurol.* 2009;**66**(12):1447–1455.

14. Davis HS, Rockwood K. Conceptualization of mild cognitive impairment: a review. *Int J Geriatr Psychiatry.* 2004;**19** (4):313–319.

15. Nyberg L, Lövdén M, Riklund K, Lindenberger U, Bäckman L. Memory aging and brain maintenance. *Trends Cogn Sci.* 2012;**16**(5):292–305.

16. Habib R, Nyberg L, Nilsson L-G. Cognitive and non-cognitive factors contributing to the longitudinal identification of successful older adults in the Betula study. *Neuropsychol Dev Cogn B Aging Neuropsychol Cogn.* 2007;**14**(3):257–273.

17. Ritchie K. The screening of cognitive impairment in the elderly: A critical review of current methods. *J Clin Epidemiol.* 1988;**41**(7):635–643.

18. Collie A, Maruff P, Currie J. Behavioral characterization of mild cognitive

impairment. *J Clin Exp Neuropsychol.* 2002;**24**(6):720–733.

19. Portet F, Ousset PJ, Visser PJ, et al. Mild cognitive impairment (MCI) in medical practice: a critical review of the concept and new diagnostic procedure. Report of the MCI Working Group of the European Consortium on Alzheimer's Disease. *J Neurol Neurosurg Psychiatry.* 2006;**77** (6):714–718.

20. Gauthier S, Reisberg B, Zaudig M, et al. Mild cognitive impairment. *Lancet (British edition).* 2006;**367**(9518):1262–1270.

21. Winblad B, Palmer K, Kivipelto M, et al. Mild cognitive impairment – beyond controversies, towards a consensus: report of the International Working Group on Mild Cognitive Impairment. *J Intern Med.* 2004;**256**(3):240–246.

22. Valenzuela M, Sachdev P. Brain reserve and dementia: a systematic review. *Psychol Med.* 2006;**36**(4):441–454.

23. Diamond MC, Rosenzweig MR, Bennett EL, Lindner B, Lyon L. Effects of environmental enrichment and impoverishment on rat cerebral cortex. *J Neurobiol.* 1972;**3**(1):47–64.

24. Mohammed A, Zhu S, Darmopil S, et al. Environmental enrichment and the brain. *Prog Brain Res.* 2002;**138**:109–133.

25. Katzman R. Education and the prevalence of dementia and Alzheimer's disease. *Neurology.* 1993;**43**(1):13–20.

26. Ngandu T, Strauss von E, Helkala E-L, et al. Education and dementia: what lies behind the association? *Neurology.* 2007;**69** (14):1442–1450.

27. Marx J. Preventing Alzheimer's: a lifelong commitment? *Science.* 2005;**309** (5736):864–866.

28. Schofield P. Alzheimer's disease and brain reserve. *Australasian J Ageing.* 1999;**18** (1):10–14.

29. Fratiglioni L, Paillard-Borg S, Winblad B. An active and socially integrated lifestyle in late life might protect against dementia. *Lancet Neurol.* 2004;**3** (6):343–353.

30. Snowdon D, Greiner L, Markesbery W. Linguistic ability in early life and the neuropathology of Alzheimer's disease and cerebrovascular disease. Findings from the Nun Study. *Ann NY Acad Sci.* 2000;**1**; (903):34–38.

31. Cadar D, Stephan BCM, Jagger C, et al. The role of cognitive reserve on terminal decline: a cross-cohort analysis from twoEuropean studies: OCTO-Twin, Sweden, and Newcastle 85+, UK. *Int J Geriatr Psychiatry.* 2016;**31** (6):601–610.

32. Lenehan ME, Summers MJ, Saunders NL, Summers JJ, Vickers JC. Relationship between education and age-related cognitive decline: a review of recent research. *Psychogeriatrics.* 2014;**15** (2):154–162.

33. Scarmeas N, Stern Y. Cognitive reserve: implications for diagnosis and prevention of Alzheimer's disease. *Curr Neurol Neurosci Rep. NIH Public Access.* 2004;**4** (5):374–380.

34. American Psychiatric Association. Diagnostic and Statistical Manual of Mental Disorders (DSM-5®). *American Psychiatric Pub*; 2013. 1 p.

35. Prince M, Wimo A, Guerchet M, Ali GC, Wu YT, Prina M. World Alzheimer Report 2015. The global impact of dementia. Ananalysis of prevalence, incidence, cost & trends; Alzheimer's Disease International. 2015.

36. Matthews FE, Stephan BCM, Robinson L, et al. A two decade dementia incidence comparison from the Cognitive Function and Ageing Studies I and II. *Nat Commun.* 2016; **19**;7:11398.

37. Larson EB, Yaffe K, Langa KM. New insights into the dementia epidemic. *N Engl J Med.* 2013;**369**(24):2275–2277.

38. Wu Y-T, Fratiglioni L, Matthews FE, et al. Dementia in western Europe: epidemiological evidence and implications for policy making. *Lancet Neurol.* 2015;**15** (1):116–124.

39. Prince M, Ali G-C, Guerchet M, Prina AM, Albanese E, Wu Y-T. Recent global trends in the prevalence and incidence of dementia, and survival with dementia. Alzheimer's Research & Therapy. *BioMed Central*; 2016;**8**(1):23.

40. Lobo A, Launer LJ, Fratiglioni L, et al. Prevalence of dementia and major subtypes in Europe: a collaborative study of population-based cohorts. Neurologic Diseases in the Elderly Research Group. *Neurology*. 2000;**54**(11 Suppl 5):S4–S9.

41. Zhang Y, Xu Y, Nie H, et al. Prevalence of dementia and major dementia subtypes in the Chinese populations: a meta-analysis of dementia prevalence surveys, 1980–2010. *J Clin Neurosci*. 2012;**19**(10):1333–1337.

42. Brunnström H, Gustafson L, Passant U, Englund E. Prevalence of dementia subtypes: a 30-year retrospective survey of neuropathological reports. *Arch Gerontol Geriatr*. 2009;**49**(1):146–149.

43. de Pedro-Cuesta J, Virués-Ortega J, Vega S, et al. Prevalence of dementia and major dementia subtypes in Spanish populations: a reanalysis of dementia prevalence surveys, 1990–2008. *BMC Neurol*. 2009;**9**(1):55.

44. Yusuf AJ, Baiyewu O, Sheikh TL, Shehu AU. Prevalence of dementia and dementia subtypes among community-dwelling elderly people in northern Nigeria. *Int Psychogeriatr*. 2011;**23**(3):379–386.

45. Russ TC, Batty GD, Hearnshaw GF, Fenton C. Geographical variation in dementia: systematic review with meta-analysis. *Int J Epidemiol*. 2012;**41**(4):1012–1032.

46. Chandra V, Ganguli M, Pandav R, Johnston J, Belle S, DeKosky ST. Prevalence of Alzheimer's disease and other dementias in rural India: the Indo-US study. *Neurology*. 1998;**51**(4):1000–1008.

47. Ferri C, Prince M, Brayne C, et al. Global prevalence of dementia: a Delphi consensus study. *Lancet*. 2005;**366**(9503):2112–2117.

48. Neuropathology Group. Medical Research Council Cognitive Function and Aging Study. Pathological correlates of late-onset dementia in a multicentre, community-based population in England and Wales. Neuropathology Group of the Medical Research Council Cognitive Function and Ageing Study (MRC CFAS). *Lancet*. 2001;**357**(9251):169–175.

49. Wattmo C, Londos E, Minthon L. Risk factors that affect life expectancy in Alzheimer's disease: a 15-year follow-up. *Dement Geriatr Cogn*. 2014;**38**(5–6):286–99.

50. Wolfson C, Wolfson D, Asgharian M, et al. A reevaluation of the duration of survival after the onset of dementia. *N Engl J Med*. 2001;**344**(15):1111–1116.

51. Winblad B, Amouyel P, Andrieu S, et al. Defeating Alzheimer's disease and other dementias: a priority for European science and society. *Lancet Neurology*. 2016;**15**(5):455–532.

52. Brodaty H, Seeher K, Gibson L. Dementia time to death: a systematic literature review on survival time and years of life lost in people with dementia. *Int Psychogeriatr*. 2012 ;**24**(7):1034–1045.

53. Day GS, Musiek ES, Roe CM, et al. Phenotypic similarities between late-onset autosomal dominant and sporadic Alzheimer disease: a single-family case-control study. *JAMA*. 2016;**73**(9):1125–1132.

54. Chang KJ, Hong CH, Lee KS, et al. Mortality risk after diagnosis of early-onset Alzheimer's disease versus late-onset Alzheimer's disease: a propensity score matching analysis. *J Alzheimers Dis*. 2017;**56**(4):1341–1348.

55. Hardy JA, Higgins GA. Alzheimer's disease: the amyloid cascade hypothesis. *Science*. 1992;**256**(5054):184–185.

56. Herrup K. The case for rejecting the amyloid cascade hypothesis. *Nat Neurosci*. 2015;**18**(6):794–799.

57. Lee H-G, Casadesus G, Zhu X, Takeda A, Perry G, Smith MA. Challenging the amyloid cascade hypothesis: senile plaques and amyloid-β as protective adaptations to Alzheimer disease. *Ann NY Acad Sci*. 2004;**1019**(1):1–4.

58. Hardy J, Selkoe D. The amyloid hypothesis of Alzheimer's disease: progress and problems on the road to therapeutics. *Science*. 2002;**297**(5580):353–356.

59. Dubois B, Hampel H, Feldman HH, et al. Preclinical Alzheimer's disease: definition, natural history, and diagnostic criteria. *Alzheimers Dement*. 2016;**12**(3):292–323.

60. Querfurth HW, LaFerla FM. Alzheimer's disease. *N Engl J Med.* 2010 ;**362** (4):329–344.

61. Schneider LS, Mangialasche F, Andreasen N, et al. Clinical trials and late-stage drug development for Alzheimer's disease: an appraisal from 1984 to 2014. *J Intern Med.* 2014;**275**(3):251–283.

62. Rönnlund M, Sundström A, Adolfsson R, Nilsson L-G. Subjective memory impairment in older adults predicts future dementia independent of baseline memory performance: Evidence from the Betula prospective cohort study. *Alzheimers Dement.* 2015;**11**(11):1385–1392.

63. Studart Neto A, Nitrini R. Subjective cognitive decline: the first clinical manifestation of Alzheimer's disease? *Dement Neuropsychol.* 2016;**10**(3):170–177.

64. Jorm AF. The Informant Questionnaire on Cognitive Decline in the Elderly (IQCODE): a review. *Int Psychogeriatr.* 2004 ;**16**(3):275–293.

65. Quinn TJ, Fearon P, Noel-Storr AH, Young C, McShane R, Stott DJ. Informant Questionnaire on Cognitive Decline in the Elderly (IQCODE) for the diagnosis of dementia within community dwelling populations. Quinn TJ, editor. *Cochrane Database Syst Rev.* 2014;**24**(4):CD010079.

66. Harrison JK, Stott DJ, McShane R, Noel-Storr AH, Swann-Price RS, Quinn TJ. Informant Questionnaire on Cognitive Decline in the Elderly (IQCODE) for the early diagnosis of dementia across a variety of healthcare settings. Quinn TJ, editor. *Cochrane Database Syst Rev.* 2016;**11**(10): CD011333.

67. Phung TKT, Chaaya M, Asmar K, et al. Performance of the 16-Item Informant Questionnaire on Cognitive Decline for the Elderly (IQCODE) in an Arabic-speaking older population. *Dement Geriatr Cogn.* 2015;**40**(5–6):276–289.

68. Gifford KA, Liu D, Lu Z, et al. The source of cognitive complaints predicts diagnostic conversion differentially among nondemented older adults. *Alzheimers Dement.* 2014;**10**(3):319–327.

69. Dubois B, Feldman HH, Jacova C, et al. Advancing research diagnostic criteria for Alzheimer's disease: the IWG-2 criteria. *Lancet Neurology.* 2014;**13**(6):614–629.

70. Ferreira D, Perestelo-Pérez L, Westman E, Wahlund L-O, Sarría A, Serrano-Aguilar P. Meta-review of CSF core biomarkers in Alzheimer's disease: the state-of-the-art after the New Revised Diagnostic Criteria. *Front Aging Neurosci.* 2014;**6**(Suppl. 179):47.

71. Rovio S, Kåreholt I, Helkala E-L, et al. Leisure-time physical activity at midlife and the risk of dementia and Alzheimer's disease. *Lancet Neurol.* 2005;**4** (11):705–711.

72. Qiu C, De Ronchi D, Fratiglioni L. The epidemiology of the dementias: an update. *Curr Opin Psychiatry.* 2007;**20** (4):380–385.

73. Kuiper JS, Zuidersma M, Oude Voshaar RC, et al. Social relationships and risk of dementia: a systematic review and meta-analysis of longitudinal cohort studies. *Ageing Res Rev.* 2015;**22**:39–57.

74. Tangney CC, Li H, Wang Y, et al. Relation of DASH- and Mediterranean-like dietary patterns to cognitive decline in older persons. *Neurology.* 2014;**83** (16):1410–1416.

75. Kivipelto M, Helkala E-L, Laakso MP, et al. Midlife vascular risk factors and Alzheimer's disease in later life: longitudinal, population based study. *BMJ.* 2001;**322**(7300):1447–1451.

76. Cheng G, Huang C, Deng H, Wang H. Diabetes as a risk factor for dementia and mild cognitive impairment: a meta-analysis of longitudinal studies. *Intern Med J.* 2012;**42**(5):484–491.

77. Kivipelto M, Kivipelto M, Ngandu T, et al. Obesity and vascular risk factors at midlife and the risk of dementia and Alzheimer disease. *Arch Neurol.* 2005;**62** (10):1556–1560.

78. Hassing LB, Dahl AK, Thorvaldsson V, et al. Overweight in midlife and risk of dementia: a 40-year follow-up study. *Int J Obesity.* 2009;**33**(8):893–898.

79. Wilson RS, Krueger KR, Arnold SE, et al. Loneliness and risk of Alzheimer disease. *Arch Gen Psychiatry.* 2007;**64**(2):234–240.

80. Cacioppo JT, Hawkey LC. Perceived social isolation and cognition. *Trends Cogn Sci.* 2009;**13**(10):447–454.

81. Ownby R, Crocco E, Acevedo A, John V, Loewenstein D. Depression and risk for Alzheimer disease – systematic review, meta-analysis, and metaregression analysis. *Arch Gen Psychiatry.* 2006 ;**63**(5):530–538.

82. Håkansson K, Soininen H, Winblad B, Kivipelto M. Feelings of hopelessness in midlife and cognitive health in later life: a prospective population-based cohort study. *PLoS ONE.* 2015;**10**(10):e0140261.

83. Håkansson K, Soininen H, Winblad B, Kivipelto M. Correction: feelings of hopelessness in midlife and cognitive health in later life: a prospective population-based cohort study. *PLoS ONE.* 2015;**10**(11):e0142465.

84. Johansson L, Guo X, Waern M, et al. Midlife psychological stress and risk of dementia: a 35-year longitudinal population study. *Brain.* 2010;**133**(8):2217–2224.

85. Sindi S, Hagman G, Håkansson K, et al. Midlife work-related stress increases dementia risk in later life: the CAIDE 30-Year Study. *J Gerontol, Series B.* 2016;**72**(6):1044–1053.

86. Luchsinger JA, Lehtisalo J, Lindström J, et al. Cognition in the Finnish diabetes prevention study. *Diabetes Res Clin Pract.* 2015;**108**(3):e63–e66.

87. Kivipelto M, Rovio S, Ngandu T, et al. Apolipoprotein E epsilon4 magnifies lifestyle risks for dementia: a population-based study. *J Cell Mol Med.* 2008;**12**(6B):2762–2771.

88. Håkansson K, Rovio S, Helkala E-L, et al. Association between mid-life marital status and cognitive function in later life: population based cohort study. *BMJ.* 2009;**339**:b2462.

89. Ewbank DC. The APOE gene and differences in life expectancy in Europe. *J Gerontol, Series A.* 2004;**59**(1):16–20.

90. Farrer LA, Cupples LA, Haines JL, et al. Effects of age, sex, and ethnicity on the association between apolipoprotein E genotype and Alzheimer disease. A meta-analysis. *JAMA.* 1997;**278**(16):1349–1356.

91. Filippini N, MacIntosh BJ, Hough MG, et al. Distinct patterns of brain activity in young carriers of the APOE-epsilon4 allele. *Proc Natl Acad Sci USA.* 2009;**106**(17):7209–7214.

92. Huang Y. Mechanisms linking apolipoprotein E isoforms with cardiovascular and neurological diseases. *Curr Opin Lipidol.* 2010;**21**(4):337–345.

93. Forsell Y, Corder E, Basun H, Lannfelt L, Viitanen M, Winblad B. Depression and dementia in relation to apolipoprotein E polymorphism in a population sample age 75. *Biol Psychiatry.* 1997;**42**(10):898–903.

94. McCarron MO, Delong D, Alberts MJ. APOE genotype as a risk factor for ischemic cerebrovascular disease: a meta-analysis. *Neurology.* 1999;**53**(6):1308–1311.

95. Gatz M, Reynolds C, Fratiglioni L, et al. Role of genes and environments for explaining Alzheimer disease. *Arch Gen Psychiatry.* 2006;**63**(2):168–174.

96. Tolppanen A-M, Solomon A, Soininen H, Kivipelto M. Midlife vascular risk factors and Alzheimer's disease: evidence from epidemiological studies. *J Alzheimers Dis.* 2012;**32**(3):531–540.

97. Amieva H, Le Goff M, Millet X, et al. Prodromal Alzheimer's disease: successive emergence of the clinical symptoms. *Ann Neurology.* 2008;**64**(5):492–498.

98. Bäckman L. Memory and cognition in preclinical dementia: what we know and what we do not know. *Can J Psychiatry.* 2008;**53**(6):354–360.

99. Jack CR, Knopman DS, Jagust WJ, et al. Hypothetical model of dynamic biomarkers of the Alzheimer's

pathological cascade. *Lancet Neurol.* 2010;**9**(1):119–128.

100. Plassman BL, Williams JW, Burke JR, Holsinger T, Benjamin S. Systematic review: factors associated with risk for and possible prevention of cognitive decline in later life. *Ann Intern Med.* 2010;**153**(3):182–193.

101. Rebok GW, Ball K, Guey LT, et al. Ten-year effects of the advanced cognitive training for independent and vital elderly cognitive training trial on cognition and everyday functioning in older adults. *J Am Geriatr Soci.* 2014;**62**(1):16–24.

102. Hill NTM, Mowszowski L, Naismith SL, Chadwick VL, Valenzuela M, Lampit A. Computerized cognitive training in older adults with mild cognitive impairment or dementia: a systematic review and meta-analysis. *Am J Psychiatry.* 2017;**174**(4):329–340.

103. Gates N, Fiatarone Singh MA, Sachdev PS, Valenzuela M. The effect of exercise training on cognitive function in older adults with mild cognitive impairment: a meta-analysis of randomized controlled trials. *Am J Geriatr Psychiatry.* 2013;**21**(11):1086–1097.

104. Groot C, Hooghiemstra AM, Raijmakers PGHM, et al. The effect of physical activity on cognitive function in patients with dementia: a meta-analysis of randomized control trials. *Ageing Res Rev.* 2016;**25**:13–23.

105. Jones L, Lambert J-C, Wang L-S, et al. Convergent genetic and expression data implicate immunity in Alzheimer's disease. *Alzheimers Dement.* 2015;**11**(6):658–671.

106. Zhu X, Yin S, Lang M, He R, Li J. The more the better? A meta-analysis on effects of combined cognitive and physical intervention on cognition in healthy older adults. *Ageing Res Rev.* 2016;**31**:67–79.

107. Ngandu T, Lehtisalo J, Solomon A, et al. A 2 year multidomain intervention of diet, exercise, cognitive training, and vascular risk monitoring versus control to prevent cognitive decline in at-risk elderly people (FINGER):a randomised controlled trial. *Lancet.* 2015;**385**(9984):1–9.

108. Andrieu S, Guyonnet S, Coley N, et al. Effect of long-term omega 3 polyunsaturated fatty acid supplementation with or without multidomain intervention on cognitive function in elderly adults with memory complaints (MAPT): a randomised, placebo-controlled trial. *Lancet Neurology.* 2017;**16**(5):377–389.

109. Moll van Charante EP, Richard E, Eurelings LS, et al. Effectiveness of a 6-year multidomain vascular care intervention to prevent dementia (preDIVA): a cluster-randomised controlled trial. *Lancet.* 2016;**388**(10046):797–805.

110. Kivipelto M, Solomon A, Ahtiluoto S, et al. The Finnish Geriatric Intervention Study to Prevent Cognitive Impairment and Disability (FINGER): Study design and progress. *Alzheimers Dement.* 2013;**9**(6):657–665.

111. Kivipelto M, Ngandu T, Laatikainen T, Winblad B, Soininen H, Tuomilehto J. Risk score for the prediction of dementia risk in 20 years among middle aged people: a longitudinal, population-based study. *Lancet Neurology.* 2006;**5**(9):735–741.

112. Richard E, Van den Heuvel E, Moll van Charante EP, et al. Prevention of dementia by intensive vascular care (PreDIVA): a cluster-randomized trial in progress. *Alz Dis Assoc Dis.* 2009 Jul;**23**(3):198–204.

113. Brookmeyer R, Kawas CH, Abdallah N, Paganini-Hill A, Kim RC, Corrada MM. Impact of interventions to reduce Alzheimer's disease pathology on the prevalence of dementia in the oldest-old. *Alzheimers Dement.* 2016;**12**(3):225–232.

114. Jorm AF, Dear KBG, Burgess NM. Projections of future numbers of dementia cases in Australia with and without prevention. *Aust NZ J Psychiatry.* 2005;**11**(12):959–963.

Cognitive Decline in Transient Ischemic Attacks or Minor Strokes

Antonia Nucera, Mahmoud Reza Azarpazhooh, and Vladimir Hachinski

Introduction

Transient ischemic attacks (TIA) and minor strokes offer an immediate and great opportunity to prevent disabling strokes, myocardial infarction, and death and decrease the chances of developing dementia. The terms "transient," "attack," "minor," and "warning" that we use every day in our clinics may lead to the idea for both professionals and patients, that symptoms are really "transient," "attack," and "minor" or at the best case scenario, they are simply a "warning." However, several studies showed that TIA and stroke, irrespective of severity and duration of symptoms, may not only lead to stroke recurrences, but also to myocardial infarctions. In addition, many patients with TIA referred to outpatient neurology/stroke prevention clinics, may only be assessed for their focal deficit, i.e., speech problems, weakness, without any assessment of cognitive abilities. In fact, these patients may have/develop cognitive decline, particularly with executive dysfunctions, and eventually may suffer a frank dementia.

Finally, acute and short period of symptoms in TIA should be differentiated from many similar paroxysmal disorders, such as migraine, the hyperventilation syndrome, seizures, and positional vertigo. Clinicians have frequently experienced a challenging time in diagnosing such stroke mimics. The accurate diagnosis of TIA, subsequent implementation and consequently the best prevention strategies are vital for patients; a misdiagnosis may cause unnecessary stress and cost for patients and their family members.

This chapter provides a brief review of definitions and clinical assessments of TIA and minor stroke and their relationship with cognitive decline.

Definitions and Clinical Importance

TIA was originally defined as a sudden onset of focal neurologic symptoms and/or signs due to transient focal brain ischemia, lasting less than 24 hours.[1,2] Although this was a practical approach, particularly in epidemiological studies, the arbitrary 24-hour time cutoff has led to the underestimation of the chance of pathological lesions in the brain. In fact, in 30 percent to 50 percent of individuals classified clinically as TIA, brain injuries were found on diffusion-weighted magnetic resonance imaging (MRI).[3,4] With the advent of modern neuroimaging techniques and their widespread usage, the definition of TIA has changed from a merely clinical and time-based classification to a tissue-based definition. TIA is currently defined as any transient episode of neurological dysfunction caused by focal brain, or retinal ischemia, without acute infarction.[4]

The definition of minor stroke is even more challenging. Although it can be clinically applied to any cases with mild and/or nondisabling symptoms, there is no general consensus for the meaning of mild and nondisabling.[5] Many studies classified their participants according to clinical symptoms, i.e., only motor or sensory deficits, or based on the severity of stroke measured by the National Institutes of Health Stroke Scale (NIHSS). Not surprisingly, final outcomes of minor stroke may vary significantly based on the definition method. Nevertheless, in a daily-based clinical practice, it is important for clinicians to diagnose subtle focal neurologic deficits due to minor strokes and differentiate them from stroke mimics.

TIA and minor strokes can dramatically increase the risk of subsequent strokes, myocardial infarctions, and death. The annual risk of stroke after TIAs and minor strokes varies from 5 percent to 15 percent depending on patient characteristics and the management strategies of stroke.[6–9] Large cohort population-based studies showed a relatively high short-term risk of stroke, particularly in the first three months after the index events (about 10 percent), with half occurring within the first two days.[4,10–13] In one neuroimaging study, although clinically symptomatic recurrences occurred in 2 percent of patients during the first week after strokes, diffusion-weighted imaging showed new lesions outside initial perfusion deficit in 15 percent of patients.[14] TIA can also significantly increase the chance of other vascular events,[15] particularly coronary artery diseases.[16] Despite the importance of the urgent treatment of TIA,[17–20] many cases with TIA, even those at the highest risk, have not received adequate treatments. Therefore, a well-designed strategy for diagnosis, classification, and management of TIA and minor strokes is an urgent priority for each and every society. In recent decades, and particularly in high-income countries, stroke prevention clinics have improved the acute management of TIA and minor stroke.[21] However, it seems that evaluation and management of cognitive abilities in TIA and minor stroke may still have room for further improvement.

Cognitive Decline after TIA and Minor Strokes

Despite the temporary profile and mild symptoms of TIA and minor strokes, many patients may experience cognitive and communicative decline beyond focal symptom resolution.[22,23] Long-term cohort studies of TIA considering cognitive functions are scant, and results vary dramatically. A recent meta-analysis showed that 29 to 68 percent of patients with TIA may develop mild cognitive impairment. In addition, a severe cognitive decline was reported in 8 to 22 percent of patients.[24]

The reasons and clinical characteristics of cognitive decline after a TIA have also not been clearly described. The explanation of a cognitive decline in TIA and minor stroke is difficult, as by definition there are no tissue-based ischemic lesions in TIA or only limited insults can be found in minor strokes. A progressive decline after TIA may be attributed to vascular risk factors, namely hypertension and diabetes, and depressive symptoms among patients.[25] Moreover, clinically silent new brain lesions after TIA may also affect cognition.[26]

It was shown that the affected domains in TIA are similar to the vascular cognitive impairment profile, with more prevalent executive dysfunction.[27] In a study of 140 patients with TIA and minor stroke, a majority of patients (57 percent) had an obvious impairment in >= 1 cognitive domains, with a relatively high prevalence of executive dysfunctions.[28] Unfortunately, many clinicians do not often assess the cognitive function in patients with TIA and minor strokes. More important, despite a widespread use of the Mini Mental State Examination (MMSE), this screening instrument is not sensitive to detect cognitive declines in patients with TIA and minor stroke.[28] Therefore, many cases with cognitive decline may remain undiagnosed, affecting the quality of life of patients.

Clinical Evaluations of TIA and Minor Strokes

The eye sees only what the mind is prepared to comprehend.
William Robertson Davies, *famous Canadian novelist*

The first step in the clinical assessment of patients in emergency rooms and outpatient clinics is a thorough clinical history. Along with a well-focused neurological examination, clinicians can formulate the combination of patient's symptoms and signs to a specific neurologic syndrome (syndrome diagnosis), localize brain lesions (anatomic localization), define etiology, and plan for further assessments considering functional outcomes.

Despite the undeniable role of neuroimaging studies in evaluation of neurologic patients, the over-reliance on imaging studies such as MRI (diagnosis from Radiology), inadequate history taking is one of the major causes of misdiagnosis in neurology wards. Table 5.1 provides a brief review of common symptoms in TIA and key questions for clinical assessments.

During the first and follow-up assessments of patients with TIA and minor stroke, it is also important to assess cognitive functions. Although a majority of physicians and researchers are familiar with the MMSE as a screening instrument,[29] this test is not sensitive for diagnosis of executive dysfunctions. Nasreddine et al[30] introduced the Montreal Cognitive Assessment (MoCA) for the assessment of cognitive functions. The MoCA is able to assess eight domains of cognitive functions, including visuospatial, executive function, naming, memory, attention, language, abstraction, and orientation. A relatively accurate assessment of executive functions provides the chance to detect even cognitive impairment at early stages. Therefore, it is recommended that the MoCA be used in patients

Table 5.1 Clinical assessments of TIA and minor strokes

Common symptoms and signs	Acute motor deficit: Hemiparesis, monoparesis, facial droop Language problems: Aphasia Speech Problems: Dysarthria Acute sensory deficit: Hemisensory deficits Visual loss: Monocular or binocular Visual field deficits: Hemianopia Acute diplopia Ataxia Vertigo (rarely in isolation)
Key questions	Onset and course: Sudden versus gradual; static versus deteriorating; with exacerbations and remissions. Type of symptoms: positive versus negative Part of the body involved : localized versus more widespread Triggering factors: exercise, sleep, posture, trauma Associated symptoms: Headache, nausea or vomiting, seizure
Uncommon findings in acute stroke	Gradual onset Bitemporal hemianopia Seizure

with TIA and minor stroke. However, even the MoCA may underestimate vascular cognitive impairment.[31] In cases with more subtle impairments and a negative screening MoCA result, a 30-minute or a 60-minute battery of neuropsychological tests (National Institute for Neurological Disorders and Stroke and the Canadian Stroke Network Harmonization Vascular Cognitive Impairment Neuropsychology Protocols) are recommended.[32]

Differential Diagnosis of TIA and Minor Stroke

Acute and temporary onset-course of TIA and minor strokes may be confused with several paroxysmal disorders, such as migraine, seizure, peripheral vestibulopathy, and hyperventilation syndrome. In a two-year cohort at a single-center emergency department, about one in every five patients with an initial diagnosis of TIA had in fact, a TIA mimic.[33] Having calculated the direct and indirect costs of stroke misdiagnosis, it seems that stroke mimics may cause a huge burden on societies and more important unnecessary emotional stress on patients and their family members. This section offers a quick review of stroke mimic, emphasizing important clinical keys for accurate clinical classifications.

Seizures

Epileptic seizures and migraine attacks are the most prevalent TIA mimics.[33] After a thorough history has been taken from patients and their family members, a generalized tonic-clonic seizure can be usually differentiated from a TIA and minor stroke. Typical clinical presentation of seizure during the ictal phase (such as a lack of consciousness, fall, tongue biting, and urinary incontinence) are important clinical keys for clinical diagnosis of seizure. While a stereotyped and recurrent pattern of events is another important clinical finding of seizure, lacunar TIA due to a single penetrating vessel (capsular warning syndrome) may also have a stereotypical pattern.[34]

In contrast to generalized seizures, focal sensory or motor seizures can sometimes be quite similar to TIA. Similar to migraine, seizures can be differentiated from TIA by positive motor or sensory symptoms, such as involuntary movements. A progressive course of symptoms spreading over the patient's limbs is also helpful for an accurate clinical judgment. However, after a seizure, particularly with a secondarily generalized pattern, some patients may develop a temporary focal neurologic deficit, known as Todd's Paralysis, named after Robert Bentley Todd. The reason of Todd's paralysis has not been clearly clarified. While Todd believed that a neuronal exhaustion due to seizure activities can lead to a postictal paralysis,[35] recent studies showed the role of a transient and local postictal brain hypoperfusion in Todd's paralysis.[36] The sequence of events, namely prodromal, preictal (immediately before the event), postictal (immediately after the event), and interictal (between the events) should be taken into account for a correct clinical diagnosis.

Finally, while a post-stroke seizure is a relatively common complication among stroke survivors,[37] during the acute phase of stroke, seizures may happen rarely, except in the patients with cerebral venous thrombosis. In addition, some patients with carotid stenosis may present with an involuntary motor movement in the ipsilateral limbs known as a shaking TIA.[38,39] This type of TIA is quite important as it can be frequently confused with a focal motor seizure. More important, a limb-shaking TIA happens usually in patients with severe large artery disease requiring an urgent vascular intervention. A simple clinical examination for a carotid bruit and further vascular imaging studies are highly recommended to diagnose a limb-shaking TIA.

Migraine

Migraine is one of the most common stroke mimics in outpatient clinics and emergency rooms.[40] While the stereotypical presentation of migraine with a severe headache may differentiate it from a TIA, an aura without headache or minimal pain is a challenging diagnosis.[41] Gradual onsets of bilateral visual, sensory, motor symptoms and speech problems that cannot be localized in a specific part of the brain are key clinical presentations to differentiate migraine from TIA. These clinical findings can be explained by the cortical spreading depression over different cerebral cortex areas, subsiding usually in 30 to a maximum of 60 minutes. In addition, the bilateral and positive nature of visual symptoms, describing zigzag lines, scintillating scotomata, and flash of lights are in favor of migraine diagnosis. As a simple clinical exam, clinicians can ask their patient to close their eyes and check if they are still able to see visual symptoms (indicating a positive nature of visual aura). It is important to remember that individuals with migraine are at a higher risk of cardiovascular diseases, such as ischemic stroke.[42,43] Moreover, a TIA or stroke in a person with history of migraine may lead to a severe headache[44] and even status migrainosus.

Vestibular Disorder

Acute dizziness or giddiness is one of the most challenging complaints in emergency departments. The most important step in the assessment of this common symptom is to define the meaning of dizziness. After a thorough history taking, clinicians should determine whether this symptom is a lack of balance and coordination (i.e., ataxia), true vertigo (i.e., a feeling of rotatory and spinning movements), or a lightheadedness. While lightheadedness can usually be attributed to nonurgent conditions such as neurometabolic or endocrine diseases, an episode of acute ataxia usually needs urgent attention and admission. However, clinicians frequently face a difficult time to differentiate a true vertigo due to stroke (central vertigo) from those attributable to vestibular disease (peripheral vertigo). Some useful clinical hints to differentiate peripheral from central vertigo are summarized in Table 5.2.

Transient Global Amnesia

Transient global amnesia (TGA) is a sudden and temporary loss of anterograde episodic memory. A lack of recall for recent events may lead to disorientation about time and place. Patients may start asking repetitive similar questions about time, place, and events without remembering the answers. Despite the relatively good outcomes of this condition, it is a quite traumatic event for the patients and relatives, and TGA may be misdiagnosed with a TIA or seizure.[45]

An almost similar age distribution and high rate of vascular risk factors make differentiation of TGA from TIA more difficult. A low rate of recurrence, along with a typical pattern of memory loss with repetitive questions can help differentiate this condition from epilepsy and stroke. Memory loss in TIA may happen very seldom due to bilateral medial temporal ischemia, and in contrast to TGA, in complex partial seizures patients may not be able to follow commands.

Amyloid Spells

Sporadic cerebral amyloid angiopathy is an age-related brain vascular disease, characterized by the beta amyloid deposition in the wall of cortical and leptomeningeal arteries.[46]

Table 5.2 Clinical differentiation between central and peripheral vertigo

Symptoms and signs	Peripheral vertigo	Central Vertigo	Clinical hints
Severity of symptoms	More severe, associated with nausea and vomiting	Less severe	Central vertigo can be severe in some cases
Tinnitus, hearing loss	More common	Rare	
Relation with position	More common	Rare	Fatigue phenomena in peripheral vertigo: the severity of symptoms may decrease with repetitive changes in positions.
Nystagmus	Horizontal, rotatory	Horizontal, vertical	Difficult to differentiate
Limb ataxia	Negative	Highly suggestive	Specific for the central type
Speech problem: dysarthria	Negative	Highly suggestive	Specific for the central type

The typical presentations include recurrent lobar intracerebral hemorrhages associated with a cognitive decline in the elderly. In addition, a transient episode of focal neurologic deficits, known as amyloid spells, has been also described. The recurrent and temporary onset of this condition as well as a gradual evolution and resolving (over seconds to minutes) of both positive and negative symptoms make this diagnosis quite challenging. Due to a high rate of lobar hemorrhage, particularly in those treated with antithrombotic medications, blood-sensitive MRI sequences (i.e., gradient echo T2-weighted MRI) is highly recommended in any suspected cases.[47]

Structural Brain Lesions

Some space-occupying lesions (SOL) in the brain, such as tumors (particularly meningiomas) and subdural hemorrhage can mimic TIA-like symptoms.[48–50] The reason for temporary focal neurologic deficits is not quite clear and might be related to partial and local cerebral blood flow impairment. A history of trauma and symptoms of raised intracranial pressure are in favor of SOL. Moreover, a widespread use of neuroimaging techniques in patients with focal neurologic deficit has led to an accurate diagnosis of SOL.

Hypoglycemia

Hypoglycemia (a blood glucose < 45 mg/dl) can result in TIA-like symptoms. Common neurological presentations include aphasia, hemiplegia, and diminished level of consciousness.[51,52] A previous history of diabetes and widespread use of rapid and bedside glucose testing make this important diagnosis easy. The immediate administration of intravenous glucose is highly recommended to treat hypoglycemia and prevent permanent neurologic squeal.

Hyperventilation Syndrome

The hyperventilation syndrome (HVS) is commonly seen in outpatient clinics. It describes a collection of usually recurrent symptoms, including sensory complaints, lightheadedness, and dyspnea with a gradual onset course.[53] After World War II and based on medical experiences during the war, Alexander Winter (1908–1978) suggested breathing into a paper bag to control HVS.[54] Although this is not currently an accepted approach for the treatment of HVS, this simple method showed the possible physiological effect of changes in the CO_2 level in the pathogenesis of symptoms. However, many well-established cases have a normal level of arterial CO_2[53], and several other factors such as neuronal hyperexcitability, respiratory alkalosis, and alteration of serum albumin/calcium have been suggested to explain HVS.

A wide range of symptoms and lack of specific diagnostic tests encouraged some authors to consider HVS as a *scientifically untenable concept.*[55,56]

Based on our experience, many patients with multiple recurrent symptoms may have HVS. Although a positive hyperventilation provocation test may be seen in normal individuals, a positive test along with gradual onset of symptoms, including lightheadedness, numbness and tingling on both sides of the patient's body, a recurrent pattern without any organic cause, and the improvement of symptoms with breath holding may indicate HVS and differentiate it from other paroxysmal disorders, particularly TIA. It is important to avoid any suggestion during the test to the patient. For example, instead of asking "do you feel numbness, tingling, or lightheadedness?" it is recommended to ask "how are you feeling?" Clinicians should record the time and duration of symptoms and then ask their patient to compare the severity of symptoms during the test with their previous presentations. It is also important to follow any cases with a possible diagnosis of HVS to prove a favorable outcome and rule out other neurologic disorders.

Summary

TIA and minor strokes are common vascular disorders that can be easily confused with several stroke mimics. Unfortunately the terms "transient" and "minor" have led to the common belief that these conditions by themselves are temporary or minor. An accurate clinical diagnosis and management of vascular risk factors can not only decrease the chance of subsequent stroke recurrences and myocardial infarction, but also decrease the chance of vascular cognitive impairment. A regular follow-up of patients with TIA and minor stroke and cognitive assessment are highly recommended.

References

1. Levy DE. How transient are transient ischemic attacks? *Neurology.* 1988;**38**:674–677.

2. Caplan LR. Transient ischemic attack: definition and natural history. *Curr Atheroscler. Rep.* 2006;**8**:276–280.

3. Brazzelli M, Chappell FM, Miranda H, et al. Diffusion-weighted imaging and diagnosis of transient ischemic attack. *Ann Neurol.* 2014;**75**:67–76.

4. Easton JD, Saver JL, Albers GW, et al. American Heart Association, American Stroke Association Stroke Council, Council on Cardiovascular Surgery and Anesthesia, Council on Cardiovascular Radiology and

Intervention, Council on Cardiovascular Nursing, Interdisciplinary Council on Peripheral Vascular Disease. Definition and evaluation of transient ischemic attack: a scientific statement for healthcare professionals from the American Heart Association/American Stroke Association Stroke Council; Council on Cardiovascular Surgery and Anesthesia; Council on Cardiovascular Radiology and Intervention; Council on Cardiovascular Nursing; and the Interdisciplinary Council on Peripheral Vascular Disease. *Stroke: J Cereb Circ.* 2009;**40**:2276–2293.

5. Fischer U, Baumgartner A, Arnold M, et al. What is a minor stroke? *Stroke: J Cereb Circ.* 2010;**41**:661–666.

6. Lovett JK, Dennis MS, Sandercock PAG, Bamford J, Warlow CP, Rothwell PM. Very early risk of stroke after a first transient ischemic attack. *Stroke: J Cereb Circ.* 2003;**34**:e138–e140.

7. Lisabeth LD, Ireland JK, Risser JMH, et al. Stroke risk after transient ischemic attack in a population-based setting. *Stroke: J Cereb Circ.* 2004;**35**: 1842–1846.

8. Kleindorfer D, Panagos P, Pancioli A, et al. Incidence and short-term prognosis of transient ischemic attack in a population-based study. *Stroke: J Cereb Circ.* 2005;**36**:720–723.

9. Coull AJ, Lovett JK, Rothwell PM, Oxford Vascular Study. Population based study of early risk of stroke after transient ischaemic attack or minor stroke: implications for public education and organisation of services. *BMJ.* 2004;**328**(7435):326.

10. Chang E Bullard MJ. Prognosis of patients discharged from the emergency department with a diagnosis of transient ischemic attack. *CJEM.* 2015;**3**(4):313–4.

11. Eliasziw M, Kennedy J, Hill MD, Buchan AM, Barnett HJM, North American Symptomatic Carotid Endarterectomy Trial Group. Early risk of stroke after a transient ischemic attack in patients with internal carotid artery disease. *Can Med Assoc J.* 2004;**170**:1105–1109.

12. Hill MD, Yiannakoulias N, Jeerakathil T, Tu JV, Svenson LW, Schopflocher DP. The high risk of stroke immediately after transient ischemic attack: a population-based study. *Neurology.* 2004;**62**:2015–2020.

13. Gladstone DJ. Management and outcomes of transient ischemic attacks in Ontario, *Can Med Assoc J.* 2004;**170**:1099–1104.

14. Kang D-W, Latour LL, Chalela JA, Dambrosia J, Warach S. Early ischemic lesion recurrence within a week after acute ischemic stroke. *Ann. Neurol.* 2003;**54**:66–74.

15. Van Wijk I, Keppelle LJ, Ginjn J Van, Windish R. Long-term survival and vascular event risk after transient ischemic attack or minor ischemic stroke: a cohort study. *J Emerg Med.* 2006;**30**:249–250.

16. McGregor A, Panagos P, Reinert S. Very early risk of a significant cardiac event after a transient ischemic attack or acute ischemic stroke. *Ann Emerg Med.* 2004:**44**:120.

17. Rothwell PM, Giles MF, Chandratheva A, et al. Effect of urgent treatment of transient ischaemic attack and minor stroke on early recurrent stroke: a prospective population-based sequential comparison. Lancet. 370(9596):1432–42;**2007**.

18. Kennedy J, Hill MD, Ryckborst KJ, Eliasziw M., Demchuk AM, Buchan AM, FASTER Investigators. Fast assessment of stroke and transient ischaemic attack to prevent early recurrence (FASTER): a randomised controlled pilot trial. *Lancet. Neurol.* 2007;**6**:961–969.

19. Elkind M. Faculty of 1000 evaluation for Fast assessment of stroke and transient ischaemic attack to prevent early recurrence (FASTER): a randomised controlled pilot trial. *F1000 – Post-publication peer review of the biomedical literature .* 30-Apr–2008.

20. Lavallée PC, Meseguer E, Abboud H, et al. A transient ischaemic attack clinic with round-the-clock access (SOS-TIA): feasibility and effects. *Lancet. Neurol.* 2007;**6**:953–960.

21. Webster F, Saposnik G, Kapral MK, Fang J, O'Callaghan C, Hachinski V. Organized

outpatient care: stroke prevention clinic referrals are associated with reduced mortality after transient ischemic attack and ischemic stroke. *Stroke: J Cereb Circ.* 2011;**42**:3176–3182.

22. Pendlebury ST, Wadling S, Silver LE, Mehta Z, Rothwell PM. Transient cognitive impairment in TIA and minor stroke. *Stroke: J Cereb Circ.* 2011;**42**: 3116–3121.

23. Fens M, van Heugten CM, Beusmans GHMI, et al. Not as transient: patients with transient ischaemic attack or minor stroke experience cognitive and communication problems; an exploratory study. *Eur J Gen Pract.* 2013;**19**:11–16.

24. van Rooij FG, Kessels RPC, Richard E, De Leeuw F-E, van Dijk EJ. Cognitive impairment in transient ischemic attack patients: a systematic review. *Cerebrovasc Dis.* 2016;**42**:1–9.

25. Prins ND. Cerebral small-vessel disease and decline in information processing speed, executive function and memory. *Brain.* 2005;2034–41.

26 Vermeer SE, Prins ND, den Heijer T, Hofman A, Koudstaal PJ, Breteler MMB. Silent brain infarcts and the risk of dementia and cognitive decline. *N Engl J Med.* 2003;**348**:1215–1222.

27. Van Rooij FG, Schaapsmeerders P, Maaijwee NAM. Persistent cognitive impairment after transient ischemic attack. *J Vasc Surg.* 2014;Stroke. 2014;**45**:2270–2274.

28. Sörös P, Harnadek M, Blake T, Hachinski V, Chan R. Executive dysfunction in patients with transient ischemic attack and minor stroke. *J Neurol Sci.* 2015;**354**:17–20.

29. Folstein MF, Folstein SE, McHugh PR, "Mini-mental state": a practical method for grading the cognitive state of patients for the clinician. *J Psychiatr Res.* 1975;**12**:189–198.

30. Nasreddine ZS, Phillips NA, Bédirian, V, et al. The Montreal Cognitive Assessment, MoCA: a brief screening tool for mild cognitive impairment. *J Am Geriatr Soc.* 2005;**53**:695–699.

31. Chan E, Khan S, Oliver R, Gill SK, Werring DJ, Cipolotti L. Underestimation of cognitive impairments by the Montreal Cognitive Assessment (MoCA) in an acute stroke unit population. *J Neurol Sci.* 2014;**343**:176–179.

32. Hachinski V, Iadecola C, Petersen RC, et al. National Institute of Neurological Disorders and Stroke-Canadian Stroke Network vascular cognitive impairment harmonization standards. *Stroke: J Cereb Circ.* 2006;**37**:2220–2241.

33. Amort M, Fluri F Schäfer J, et al. Transient ischemic attack versus transient ischemic attack mimics: frequency, clinical characteristics and outcome. *Cerebrovasc Dis.* 2011;**32**:57–64.

34. Donnan GA, O'Malley HM, Quang L, Hurley S, Bladin PF. The capsular warning syndrome: pathogenesis and clinical features. *Neurology.* 1993;**43**:957–962.

35. Todd RB. Clinical lectures on paralysis, certain diseases of the brain, and other affections of the nervous system. London, 1856.

36. Mathews MS, Smith WS, Wintermark M, Dillon WP, Binder DK. Local cortical hypoperfusion imaged with CT perfusion during postictal Todd's paresis. *Neuroradiology.* 2008;**50**:397–401.

37. Forsgren L, Bucht G, Eriksson S, Bergmark L. Incidence and clinical characterization of unprovoked seizures in adults: a prospective population-based study. *Epilepsia.* 1996;**37**:224–229.

38. Baquis GD, Pessin MS, Scott RM. Limb shaking–a carotid TIA. *Stroke: J Cereb Circ.* 1985;**16**:444–448.

39. Abe K, Suda S. Limb-shaking TIA: cortical myoclonus associated with ICA stenosis. *Neurology.* 2016;**86**(3):307–9.

40. Bruno EC. Variables associated with discordance between emergency physician and neurologist diagnoses of transient ischemic attacks in the emergency department. Annal of Emergency Medicine. 2012; 5(1)19–26.

41. Fisher CM. Late-life migraine accompaniments–further experience. *Stroke: J Cereb Circ.* 1986;**17**:1033–1042.

42. Etminan M, Takkouche B, Isorna FC, Samii A. Risk of ischaemic stroke in people with migraine: systematic review and meta-analysis of observational studies. *BMJ.* 2005;1–4.

43. Schürks M, Rist PM, Bigal ME, Buring JE, Lipton RB, Kurth T. Migraine and cardiovascular disease: systematic review and meta-analysis. *BMJ.* 2009;**339**(7728): b3914.

44. Olesen J, Friberg L, Olsen TS, et al. Ischaemia-induced (symptomatic) migraine attacks may be more frequent than migraine-induced ischaemic insults. *Brain: J Neurol.* 1993;**116**(Pt 1):187–202.

45. Owen D, Paranandi B, Sivakumar R., Seevaratnam M. Classical diseases revisited: transient global amnesia. *Postgrad Med J.* 2007;**83**:236–239.

46. Charidimou A, Gang Q, Werring DJ. Sporadic cerebral amyloid angiopathy revisited: recent insights into pathophysiology and clinical spectrum. *J Neurol Neurosurg Psychiatry.* 2012;**83**:124–137.

47. Charidimou A, Baron J-C, Werring DJ. Transient focal neurological episodes, cerebral amyloid angiopathy, and intracerebral hemorrhage risk: looking beyond TIAs. *Int J Stroke : Off J Int Stroke Soc.* 2013;**8**:105–108.

48. Melamed E, Lavy S, Reches A, Sahar A. Chronic subdural hematoma simulating transient cerebral ischemic attacks. Case report. *J Neurosurg.* 1975;**42**:101–103.

49. Ueno Y, Tanaka A, Nakayama Y, Transient neurological deficits simulating transient ischemic attacks in a patient with meningioma–case report. *Neurol medico-chirurgica.* 1998;**38**:661–665.

50. Davidovitch S Gadoth N. Neurological deficit-simulating transient ischemic attacks due to intracranial meningioma: report of 3 cases. *Eur Neurol.* 1987;**28**:24–26.

51. Andrade R, Mathew V, Morgenstern MJ, et al. Hypoglycemic hemiplegic syndrome. *Ann Emerg Med.* 1984;**13**:529–531.

52. Wallis WE, Donaldson I, Scott RS, Wilson J. Hypoglycemia masquerading as cerebrovascular disease (hypoglycemic hemiplegia). *Ann Neurol.* 1985;**18**: 510–512.

53. Hirokawa Y, Kondo T, Ohta Y, Kanazawa O. Clinical characteristics and outcome of 508 patients with hyperventilation syndrome. *Nihon Kyōbu Shikkan Gakkai zasshi.* 1995;**33**:940–946.

54. Winter A. A rapid emergency treatment for hyperventilation syndrome. *J Am Med Assoc.* 1951;**147**(10):990.

55. Hornsveld H, Garssen B. Hyperventilation syndrome: an elegant but scientifically untenable concept. *Neth J Med.* 1997;**50**:13–20.

56. Bass C., Hyperventilation syndrome: a chimera? *J Psychosom Res.* 1997;**42**:421–426.

The Stroke Patient and Cognition

Michael Brainin and Yvonne Teuschl

Introduction

Disorders of cognition (neurocognitive disorders) following stroke occur between 7 percent in population-based studies of first-ever stroke patients and 41 percent in hospital-based studies that included recurrent strokes. Milder forms of cognitive deterioration following stroke are found between 22 percent and 84 percent of the time depending on definition, testing, and time of investigation. Incidence rates are 2–3 percent, increasing annually at linear rates. Importantly, milder forms can also be quite disabling and hinder rehabilitation and reuptake of occupational and social roles. Probably all stroke patients are at risk of suffering from cognitive deterioration, but some risk factors are especially important, such as location of stroke in the brain, initial stroke severity, previous strokes, level of prestroke cognition, and presence of vascular risk factors. Genetic and inflammatory biomarkers are under investigation, but observational data suggest that high levels of interleukins and C-reactive protein have predictive value. Cognitive and brain reserve can protect against cognitive deterioration. This reserve depends on education, leisure activities, and social interactions. Diagnosis of poststroke cognitive deterioration (mild neurocognitive disorder) varies according to test instruments used. Usually, a short bedside test is used, and an extended neuropsychological test battery is applied later. Variations also result from speech disturbances and emotional disorders such as depression. Computed tomography (CT) and magnetic resonance imaging (MRI) confirm the diagnosis and provide additional information on location and size of infarct, previous infarcts, white matter lesions, microbleeds, and brain atrophy. Management focuses on prevention and includes cognitive training and modification of risk factors. Lifestyle modifications have been shown to be beneficial in preventing cognitive decline in persons at risk of dementia. To date, smaller trials have not shown similar interventions to be effective in stroke patients. New studies on molecular changes invoked by social support and environmental enrichment strategies to preserve cognition are ongoing.

Prevalence, Incidence, and Natural History of Poststroke Cognitive Impairment (Neurocognitive Disorder)

Following stroke the risk of developing dementia doubles, and the progression rate from mild cognitive impairment to dementia increases. The prevalence of dementia is four to six times higher after stroke than in stroke-free persons of the same age.[1]

Prevalence

Prevalence rates of cognitive impairment in stroke survivors varies between studies depending on the setting, the population, the exclusion criteria (prestroke dementia, recurrent stroke, aphasia), the criteria used for the diagnosis of cognitive impairment, and the timing of cognitive testing.[1,2] In a systematic review by Pendlebury and Rothwell the prevalence rate of poststroke dementia in the first year after stroke ranges from 7 percent in population-based studies of first-ever stroke excluding prestroke dementia to 41 percent in hospital-based studies including recurrent stroke and prestroke dementia.[1]

The prevalence of mild cognitive impairment is difficult to assess because of the multitude of cognitive tests and definitions for cognitive impairment used in different studies. However, up to 86 percent of patients were found to have some cognitive deficits when examined within one month after stroke using sensitive neuropsychological test instruments and when assessing different cognitive domains.[3–6] In the postacute phase, ranging from 3 months to 14 years, cognitive impairment (mild cognitive deficits or dementia) was found in 22 to 84 percent of stroke patients.[5,7–12]

Incidence and Natural History

Strategic infarcts denote infarcts in brain regions critical to cognitive functioning and can immediately result in severe cognitive impairment. With infarcts in other brain locations, a delay of weeks or several months can occur before cognitive impairment becomes apparent. Furthermore, functional magnetic resonance imaging (fMRI) studies suggest that the disruption of neural connectivity in functional networks can lead to poststroke cognitive symptoms attributable to regions that are remote from the lesion site and structurally intact. Recovery of cognitive function in these regions may be possible by neural compensation through a reorganization of neuronal networks.[13,14]

The risk of poststroke dementia was found to be highest in the first months after stroke, which might partially be due to unrecognized cognitive impairment before stroke.[2] After the initial poststroke dementia peak due to infarcts in "strategic" locations, the cumulative incidence of poststroke dementia increases at a rate of 3 percent and 1.7 percent per year in hospital-based and population-based studies, respectively.[1] The longest observational period was 25 years in a population-based study that reported a cumulative incidence of poststroke dementia of 48 percent at year 25.[1]

The conversion rate of mild cognitive impairment to poststroke dementia varies depending on the definition of mild cognitive impairment. In a hospital-based cohort, the proportion of stroke patients meeting the criteria for early cognitive impairment at three months varied from 17 percent to 66 percent, depending on the criteria used; 5–11 percent of those developed dementia during the following 15 months.[15]

Up to 55 percent of patients recover from deficits identified during the acute phase of stroke. Recovery mainly happens during the first weeks[7,16–19] and may indicate a general improvement due to spontaneous recovery while specific tasks remain impaired.[20]

Whereas the majority of patients recover or remain stable, approximately one-third decline cognitively in a delayed fashion.[15,19] A prospective cohort study of 23,572 (525 incident strokes) community-dwelling adults, aged 45 or older, found that incident stroke accelerates long-term cognitive decline in global cognition and executive functions in stroke survivors but not in new learning or verbal memory compared to prestroke decline and to no-strokes.[21]

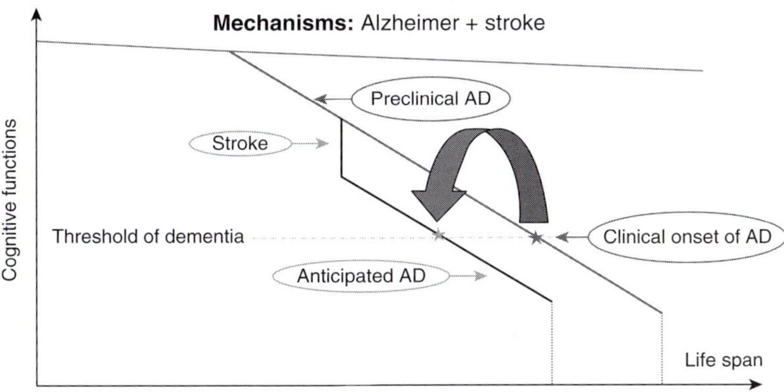

Figure 6.1 The interaction between stroke and Alzheimer's disease. In a preclinical Alzheimer's phase, cognitive functions deteriorate gradually reaching the point of clinical onset of dementia (star, right). Occurrence of stroke can unmask the dementia making it appear earlier in the life span (star, left).
Pasquier and Leys, *J Neurol.* 1997;244:135–142, with permission.

The mechanisms for this delayed onset remain unclear, but vascular as well as neuro-degenerative mechanisms are involved, and stroke seems to accelerate ongoing gradual processes of cognitive decline (Figure 6.1).[22] A number of interconnected mechanisms harming the neurovascular unit (formed from astrocytes, microglia, capillary endothelium, neurons, pericytes, and extracellular matrix) are likely to contribute to the progression of poststroke cognitive impairment.[23] Stroke leads to a breakdown of the neurovascular unit resulting in impaired cerebral blood flow regulation and blood brain barrier transport. Apart from immediate damage, this may trigger processes that started before stroke. Nevertheless, the mechanisms of delayed processes are not well understood, making the diagnosis and the treatment difficult. A recent study focusing on delayed-onset dementia by excluding patients with dementia at three to six months after stroke found that factors related to vascular disease (history of hypertension and diabetes mellitus, and imaging indicators for small vessel disease – more than three lacunes and confluent white matter changes) are independently associated with delayed-onset dementia, whereas indicators for Alzheimer disease AD (Pittsburg compound B) were only present in 19 percent of patients with delayed cognitive decline.[24]

Risk Factors

Stroke Subtypes and Imaging-Related Risk Factors

Stroke severity, infarct volume, left-hemispheric stroke, the number of previous strokes, multiple infarcts, silent infarcts, global cerebral atrophy, medial-temporal lobe atrophy, white matter changes, cerebral microbleeds, and enlarged perivascular spaces have been associated with poststroke cognitive impairment.[1,2,23,25,26]

Intracerebral and subarachnoid hemorrhages have been associated with a higher 30-year risk of poststroke dementia in a large Danish cohort.[27]

Stroke subtypes leading to more severe deficits, such as total anterior circulation infarcts, were also associated with a higher risk of cognitive impairment.[7,28] However, these subtypes are also associated with higher mortality rates, and may thus make the interpretation of cognitive deficits according to stroke subtype difficult. A recent MRI study using a voxel-based lesion-symptom mapping (VLSM) analysis found that stroke location (the number of eloquent voxels) determined 24 to 72 hours after stroke was a predictor of cognition at 3 months, independent of initial stroke severity.[29]

In a long-term community-based study, the age-standardized annual rates for cognitive impairment were relatively stable after three months poststroke, but differed in prevalence and progression according to different stroke subtypes. While the impairment rates were highest in total anterior circulation and large artery atherosclerosis infarcts, lacunar infarctions and small vessel occlusion showed a more stepwise progression.[7] This suggests progressive mechanisms in the latter subtypes. Indeed, lacunar strokes have repeatedly been associated with an increased risk for cognitive decline.[19,30] In a meta-analysis, a similar proportion of patients with lacunar and nonlacunar stroke had mild cognitive impairment or dementia up to four years after stroke.[31] Furthermore, lacunar infarcts have been associated with white matter tract abnormalities remote from the lesion visible on conventional MRI images and might thus have more widespread effects on white matter microstructure.[32] Another small MRI study suggests that silent infarcts in the basal ganglia territory may reduce global and local efficiency of the white matter network suggesting a disruption of the cortical network and leading to cognitive impairment.[33]

Thus, clinicians should be aware that despite the fact that lacunar strokes affect a small area of the brain, are often mild, and present without cognitive impairment during the acute phase, these patients are at high risk of cognitive decline.

Recurrent Stroke

A recurrent stroke more than doubles the risk for poststroke dementia. Excluding those patients that already have dementia when stroke occurs, 1 in 10 will develop dementia after a first-ever stroke whereas 1 in 3 will develop dementia following stroke recurrence.[1] Thus, secondary stroke prevention is not only important to prevent the burden of more strokes but also for the preservation of cognition.

Age

"Normal" aging is associated with structural changes in the brain and correlates with an age-related decline in cognition. Loss of synapses occurs, and cortical neurons as well as axons are lost leading to atrophy and to decrease of brain weight.[34] These "normal" changes are aggravated in poststroke cognitive impairment, leading to regional and/or diffuse atrophy and decreases in metabolism. With increased life expectancy, clinicians are more likely to be confronted with stroke cases that are accompanied by preexisting cognitive impairment.

Age is an important risk factor for dementia, and young adults (<50 years) have a better cognitive prognosis after stroke compared to elderly persons. Nevertheless, even in a relatively young population up to 50 percent of the patients showed a below-average performance after a mean follow-up time of 11 years.[35] Thus, the long-term impact of stroke on cognition should not be underestimated even in younger patients with a seemingly good prognosis, especially because cognitive deficits at young age have a major impact on working and family life.

Vascular Risk Factors

A number of treatable vascular risk factors contributing to the risk of stroke such as hypertension, dyslipidaemia, diabetes, atrial fibrillation, smoking, overweight, physical inactivity, and poor diet have been associated with an increased risk of dementia.[36–39] It is noteworthy that accumulating vascular risk factors already have measureable effects on cognitive performance. In two cohort studies, persons with an elevated ten-year risk of stroke showed significant lower performance in cognitive tests for visual-spatial memory, attention, organization, scanning, and abstract reasoning,[40] and in immediate and delayed verbal memory, semantic verbal fluency, and processing speed.[41] In cognitively normal older persons, a high cardiovascular risk at baseline was associated with greater decline in resting state cerebral blood flow in orbitofrontal, medial frontal/anterior cingulate, insular, precuneus, and brain stem regions after a mean of 7.4 years.[42]

In young patients (18–50 years) cognitive performance 14 days after stroke correlated negatively with the number of vascular risk factors.[43]

Early preventive measures targeting modifiable vascular risk factors should thus already start in high-risk persons before stroke accelerates processes leading to cognitive impairment.

Other Risk Factors (Biomarkers)

The ε4 allele of apolipoprotein E (*APOE4*) is a well-known risk factor for Alzheimer disease, and increasing evidence suggests that it may also play a role in other neurodegenerative diseases. Its association with vascular dementia and poststroke cognitive impairment is still controversial.[44]

Systemic inflammation and inflammatory markers have been associated with cognitive impairment, particularly in Alzheimer disease, but have not yet been confirmed for poststroke cognitive impairment. However, recent observational studies have suggested inter-leukin 6, interleukin 12, and C-reactive protein as predictors for poststroke cognitive impairment.[45–47]

Prestroke Cognitive Impairment

Prestroke cognitive impairment is a significant predictor for poststroke dementia.[1] However, cognitive impairment is often undiagnosed before stroke. A meta-analysis estimates the prevalence of prestroke dementia being 14 percent in hospital-based studies and 9 percent in population-based studies[1].

Cognitive decline is often already apparent before stroke, especially among individuals that do not survive stroke (see Figure 6.2).[48–50] This indicates that degenerative processes may start years before stroke.

Cognitive Reserve

The concept of brain reserve or cognitive reserve implies that some persons can tolerate more pathological changes before showing clinical symptoms of cognitive decline. Reserve is seen as a moderator between pathology and clinical outcome that may explain individual differences. Brain reserve refers to a reserve of neural substance (brain volume, neurons, synapses) that allows more pathological changes, whereas cognitive reserve refers to task performance that reduces the effects of cognitive decline in some individuals.[51]

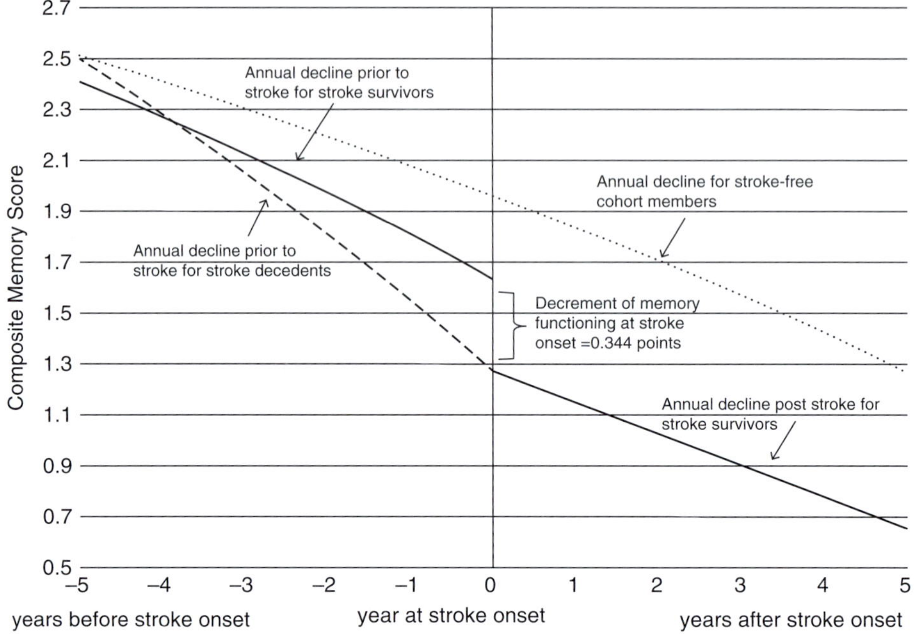

Figure 6.2 Already several years before the onset of stroke a decline of memory can be seen in comparison to a cohort that remains stroke-free. At the onset of stroke (solid vertical line at 0), the decline continues and is more severe in stroke survivors. (Trajectory of memory score for stroke survivors (n=1189) vs. stroke decedents (n=385) vs. stroke-free cohort members (n=15 766) during entire follow-up.) Capistrant, Ehntholt, Glymour, *Stroke*. 2012;43:2561–2566, with permission from Wang.

In fact, data of two longitudinal clinical-pathologic studies showed that pathologic indices of Alzheimer disease, cerebrovascular disease, and Lewy body disease were associated with faster rates of cognitive decline but nevertheless explained together only 41 percent of variation in cognitive decline, suggesting that other sources are additionally involved in late-life cognitive changes.[52]

Cognitive reserve can be built up from multiple sources and may change throughout the lifetime. Observational studies suggest that education, occupation, leisure activities, and social interactions can protect against dementia and cognitive decline.[51,53] In stroke studies, low education and premorbid intelligence were predictors for dementia.[1,54] One hospital-based cohort study showed that regular participation in intellectual activities in the year before the stroke reduced the risk for poststroke dementia.[55] In another study, bilingualism was associated with better cognitive outcome seven months poststroke.[56]

Diagnosis

The cognitive deficits observed after stroke are heterogeneous. This is due not only to methodological differences between studies and to unrecognized prestroke deficits but also to different locations, severity, and etiologies of infarcts, and to the involvement of a variety of underlying processes. Vascular cognitive impairment can affect one or several different cognitive domains; however, some domains such as executive functions or speed of mental processing are more likely to be affected.[4,5,6,10,17,20,57,58] Thus, Hachinski et al 2006 suggest that neuropsychological test batteries for vascular cognitive impairment should test for a wide range of abilities and include the four domains: executive/activation, languages, visuospatial, and memory.[59]

Test Instruments

Neuropsychological test instruments differ across studies, clinics, and countries. A survey identified 213 neuropsychological instruments used in 25 European countries to assess dementia in clinical practice.[60] In addition to availability and the need for validated versions for different languages, neuropsychological test instruments have to fulfill a number of criteria such as specific psychometric properties, usability, and time and cost constraints.[59]

In clinical practice, initial cognitive testing may be performed with a short screening tool, and an extensive neuropsychological tests battery may be used later by cognitive specialists to determine the nature and severity of potential cognitive problems in peculiar patients.

An increasing number of national stroke guidelines recommend the use of validated screening tools to detect cognitive impairment after stroke;[61] the two best known and widespread tests being the Montreal Cognitive Assessment (MoCA) and the Mini Mental State Examination (MMSE). However, based on current knowledge, no cognitive screening test has been found to be superior.[61,62] Thus, the choice of the test instrument should be based on other factors, such as the purpose of the test, clinical usability, availability of resources, patient population and time of testing.[61,62] For example, if a higher sensitivity is preferred at cost of specificity, the MoCA or the Addenbrooke's Cognitive Examination-Revised may be preferred over the MMSE. Furthermore, cut-offs can be changed to adapt sensitivity. Recently, a new domain-specific cognitive screen has been developed for stroke making it possible to include patients with aphasia and neglect.[12]

An extended test battery should assess multiple domains and be composed by validated neuropsychological tests fulfilling different criteria regarding psychometrics, usability, costs, time, language, and culture (e.g., National Institute of Neurological Disorders and Stroke–Canadian Stroke Network Vascular Cognitive Impairment Harmonization Standards Neuropsychological Battery).[59] Possible limits of an extended test battery are that it may be exhausting and time consuming for cognitively more affected patients and that most cognitive tests are not adapted for the use in aphasic patients.

Neuropsychological testing should take into account education (cognitive reserve) and age. Unfortunately, as a result of an increasing number of the "oldest-old," there is a lack of age-appropriate normative data for "normal" cognition in people aged 65+. Especially in persons with large cognitive reserve, attention should be paid to subjective complaints about deficits in activities of daily living. Subjective cognitive complaints are highly prevalent after stroke and tend to increase over time, but they are inconsistently associated with objectively measured cognitive performance and seem better at reflecting ecologically valid neuropsychological tests.[63,64]

Immediate stroke-related factors such as impairment of speech, language, hearing, vision, and psychological symptoms – especially depression and anxiety – which may influence cognitive test results, should be taken into account.

If possible prestroke cognitive impairment should be assessed retrospectively. The most commonly employed validated assessment is the Informant Questionnaire for Cognitive Decline in the Elderly (IQCODE), a proxy-rated questionnaire, in which an informant rates the change in function over the last 10 years.[65] The IQCODE is relatively unaffected by education and culture, but it is affected by informants' well-being, and the relationship between the informant and the subject.

All stroke patients are at risk of cognitive decline independent of age, stroke severity, or stroke location and should thus be considered for screening and subsequent cognitive testing once the clinical condition permits.

Imaging

Most acute stroke patients undergo CT brain imaging to exclude hemorrhages and some stroke mimics. In addition, CT provides important information on the size of the infarct, the location, old lesions, the presence and severity of white matter lesions, microbleeds, and brain atrophy – features that may predict subsequent cognitive impairment and dementia.[1,66] If not contra-indicated, MRI, rather than CT, is preferred for research and routine clinical use because it has higher sensitivity and specificity for detecting pathological changes (see Figure 6.3 for an example of MRI in a case with progressing brain atrophy coupled to cognitive deterioration).

Several MRI markers of small vessel disease (SVD) (lacunes, white matter hyperinten-sities, cerebral microbleeds, silent infarcts, white matter changes, global cerebral atrophy, medial-temporal lobe atrophy) were identified as determinants of poststroke dementia.[66] Vascular lesions include subcortical areas of the brain, especially subfrontal white matter circuits, strategic areas of single infarction such as the dominant thalamus or angular gyrus, deep frontal areas and the left hemisphere, and bilateral brain infarcts or volume-driven cortical-subcortical infarctions reaching a critical threshold of tissue loss or injury.[67] Mild to moderate stroke patients with preexisting white matter lesions are more vulnerable to cognitive impairment, regardless of their new ischemic lesions.[68] Results from SMART-MR study suggested that the interaction between brain atrophy and white matter hyper-intensities or infarcts could aggravate the cognitive decline.[69]

Management

No specific therapeutic strategy has shown convincing clinical evidence of restoring cogni-tive function or preventing its decline after stroke.[70,71] Acute treatment and early

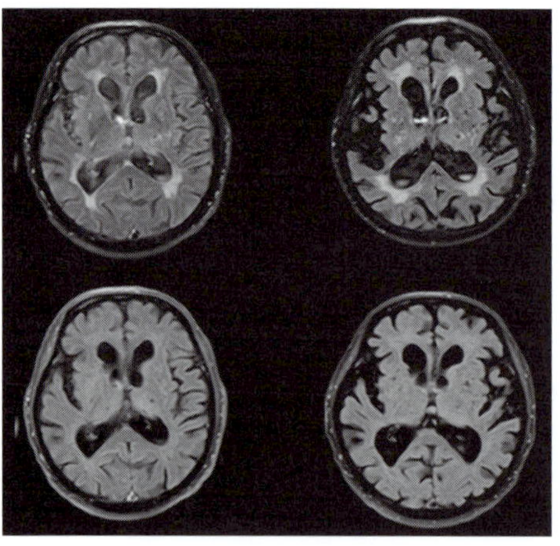

Figure 6.3a This case demonstrates the progression of brain atrophy coupled to cognitive deterioration in a patient with small vessel disease. Left row (April 2013), right row (November 2015): 72-year old male patient had suffered several small strokes previously and presented again with a new small right-sided capsular stroke in 11/2015 (Fig 6.3b). While he regained motor abilities within 10 days, his cognition deteriorated from April 2013 to November 2015. In the Mini-Mental Test Examination he had deteriorated from mild neurocognitive impairment (23/30) points to severe neurocognitive impairment (18/30). The corresponding MRI scans showed marked progression of atrophic changes, while white matter lesions and microbleeds (not shown) had only progressed minimally.

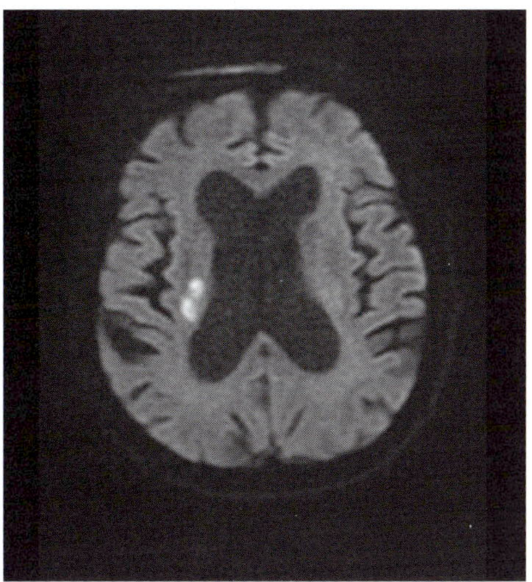

Figure 6.3b The same patient showing an acute right-sided capsular infarct on diffusion weighted MRI scan on admission (11/2015).

rehabilitation at stroke units aim at preventing further complications, to limit the damage from stroke lesions and to improve outcome.

Cognitive Training

Cognitive training during rehabilitation aims at improving specific deficits or at teaching compensation strategies to allow patients independency, participation, and the resumption of their day-to-day activities. Treatment methods differ broadly according to the theoretical basis, the design, and the components.[72,73] Cognitive training can be delivered in groups, or as individual training; it may be computer based or include the use of assistive devices such as diaries, notebooks, audiotapes, or audio alarms. Training should be adapted individually according to the goals, preferences, and individual deficits of each patient. Special attention should be paid to communication deficits and to psychological symptoms. In the case of severe deficits, caregivers should be involved to provide additional support for the patient as well as for the caregivers themselves.[61]

The evidence for the efficacy, intensity, dosage, and best method of cognitive interventions for the improvement of cognition after stroke is limited.[72,73] There is good evidence for the effectiveness of cognitive training for attention, memory, and executive functions in traumatic brain injuries, but data are insufficient for stroke.[72–76]

Pharmacotherapy

Many different treatments have been developed or tested for neuroprotection in stroke such as cerebrolysin, citicoline, actovegin, selective serotonin reuptake inhibitors, or nitric oxide donors.[70,77] However, so far none of these drugs has shown convincing evidence for the preservation of cognition after stroke.

Cholinesterase inhibitors and the N-methyl-D-aspartate (NMDA) receptor antagonist, memantine, used in Alzheimer dementia, were tested in a few short-term trials in vascular cognitive impairment showing small and mixed effects.[77] These drugs might be relevant for only a few selected patients.

Behavioral Psychological Symptoms

Behavioral and psychological symptoms such as depression, anxiety, apathy, or fatigue are often a consequence of stroke and contribute to cognitive impairment, or may influence the cognitive test results in the stressful clinical setting of acute stroke.

Approximately one-third of stroke patients develop depression, the commonest neuropsychiatric symptom[78] after stroke. Patients with stroke should be screened for depressive symptoms. There are several therapeutic strategies for poststroke depression, including both pharmacological and nonpharmacological approaches. There is some evidence supporting the use of antidepressant drugs for the improvement of depressive symptoms, but they are also associated with adverse events.[79] Furthermore, selective serotonin reuptake inhibitors (SSRIs) may be associated with overall recovery after stroke, also in patients without depression.[80] Despite a lack of data for nonpharmacological psychotherapeutic interventions as sole therapy, they may be considered because of the side effects of antidepressant drugs.

Prevention

The delayed cognitive impairment that is observed in some persons after stroke offers the chance for a therapeutic window to stop or slow down processes that may have started before stroke. In the absence of effective pharmacological interventions, multidomain interventions with rigorous control of vascular risk factors including lifestyle modification, treatment of neuropsychiatric symptoms, and provision of a cognitive and social stimulating environment may be the best opportunity to preserve cognition as long as possible.

Control of Vascular Risk Factors and Lifestyle Modifications

Modifiable vascular risk factors have repeatedly been associated with cognitive decline in observational studies. Thus, despite lack of evidence from large, well-designed randomized controlled trials, it seems plausible that established pharmacological secondary stroke prevention strategies in combination with lifestyle-oriented interventions adjusted to individual risk factors can reduce the risk of cognitive decline and dementia in stroke survivors.[70]

Interventions should be multimodal and target all individual risk factors together: these include optimal control of blood pressure, cholesterol, and blood glucose; physical activity; weight control; smoking cessation; and healthy diet.

The recently terminated Finnish Geriatric Intervention Study to Prevent Cognitive Impairment and Disability (FINGER) – a large randomized controlled trial including 1,260 people aged 60–77, who are at risk of dementia and have a cognitive performance at mean or slightly lower level than expected for their age – is the first to show that multidomain intervention (diet, exercise, cognitive training, vascular risk monitoring) compared to a control group with general health advice can improve or maintain cognitive functions after a period of two years.[81] In this trial, being at risk of dementia was determined based on a multifactorial risk score including age, hypertension, hypercholesterolemia, physical inactivity, obesity, and education. However, the Prevention of Dementia by Intensive Vascular care (preDIVA) trial, a large cluster-randomized nurse-led vascular multidomain intervention trial in elderly people, did not find any effect on cognition after six years.[82]

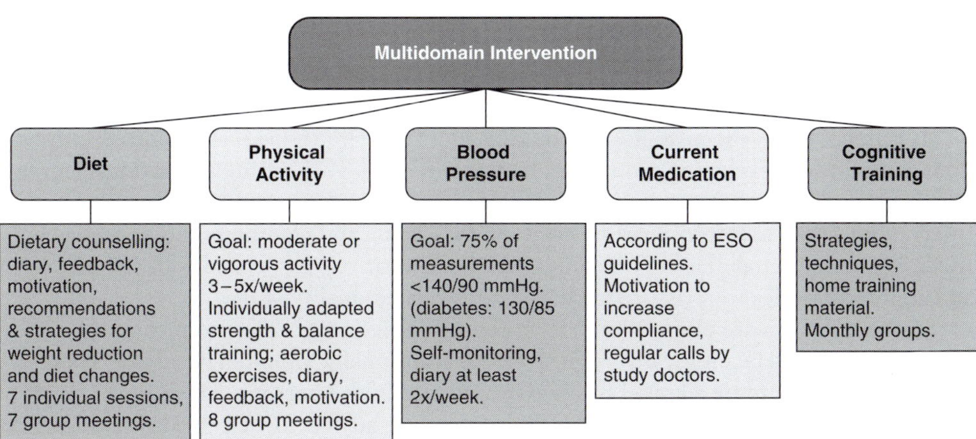

Figure 6.4 Simultaneous, multimodal interventions in the Austrian Polyintervention Study to Prevent Cognitive Decline after Ischemic Stroke.
Matz, Teuschl, Firlinger, et al. *Stroke.* 2015;46:2874–2880.

In stroke patients, only two small randomized controlled trials, with 200 patients each, tested the effect of multidomain interventions compared to standard care on poststroke cognition.[83,84] One study was based on the interventions of the FINGER study but found no differences in cognition after two years (see Figure 6.4 and reference 83). Similarly, the other study found no change in cognitive outcome after one year; however, significant positive effects were found on depressive symptoms.[84,85] However, both studies might have been underpowered.

An observational community-based study of 1682 first-ever stroke patients found that optimal management of secondary prevention therapy of vascular risk factors including anticoagulant, antiplatelet, antihypertensive, and lipid-lowering drugs was related to a lower risk of cognitive decline up to 10 years poststroke.[86] A small randomized controlled trial in 83 patients found no effect of 24 months of intensive blood pressure and lipid lowering on cognitive outcome after stroke compared to guideline treatment.[87]

Recently a large randomized controlled trial including participants with a high cardiovascular risk, aged from 55 to 80 years, showed that a Mediterranean diet supplemented with extra-virgin olive oil or nuts reduced the incidence of major cardiovascular events, including stroke, compared to a control diet (advice to reduce dietary fat). In a substudy of this trial, including 447 cognitively healthy participants, improvements were found in some cognitive tests for the two Mediterranean diet groups compared to controls after a median follow-up of 4.1 years.[88] This is the first randomized controlled trial showing beneficial effects of changes in dietary pattern on cognitive outcome.

Stroke patients are highly sedentary after stroke, and their cardiovascular fitness is reduced and lower than in age-matched controls. Furthermore, gait and balance early after stroke have been associated with cognitive function one year after stroke.[89] In addition to its positive effects on vascular factors, physical activity has repeatedly been found to be beneficial for cognition in cognitive healthy elderly people and in people with mild cognitive impairment. The evidence for stroke patients is limited; however, the available data suggests that physical activity enhances cognitive performance after stroke and may enhance brain plasticity especially when cognitive and physical exercise are combined.[90,91]

No randomized controlled trial has found evidence for effective strategies for smoking cessation in stroke patients.

In general, to be effective, lifestyle modifications require individually tailored interventions, support for developing motivation to make changes, goal-setting and action-planning, ongoing encouragement to maintain changes, and advice on how to manage relapses. Interventions have to improve self-efficacy and the coping and planning skills of participants. In stroke, several rehabilitation outcomes have been positively associated with self-efficacy,[92] and coping strategies were associated with health-related quality of life.[93]

Stroke survivors are often elderly, have comorbidities, may suffer from communication problems, and may be physically, cognitively, or emotionally impaired by stroke. Therefore interventions have to be adapted to their specific needs and barriers. These may consist of help with logistic or transport problems, structured advice to help understanding and applying instructions, social support to increase self-confidence, to improve empowerment, and to overcome depressive symptoms or individual adaptations of interventions because of health problems.[94,95] Safety concerns related to patients' medical condition (e.g., cardiac disease) might be a barrier for physiotherapists to include patients in structured aerobic exercise programs and should be addressed.[96] Finally, relatives and caregivers should be involved in lifestyle interventions to give support for behavioral changes and to help adapting patients' environment (e.g., for dietary changes).

New technologies such as internet-based tools, smartphone apps, or text messages are more and more integrated in lifestyle intervention programs.[97,98] These tools have the advantage to encourage active self-management leading to better adherence and empowerment, to offer the possibility of individualized health advice and counseling, to allow immediate feedback, to increase motivation by self-reported progress and independence in time and location at low cost without much effort from personnel. However, despite the possibility for interactive online education and group discussions, these technologies cannot replace social face-to-face interaction or physical help during exercise. Furthermore, these tools may not be suited for elderly people with cognitive impairment who are not habituated to this technology.

Enriched Environment (Cognitive, Social, and Physical Activities)

While an enriched environment was found to increase brain plasticity especially early after stroke in animal models, there is no evidence for stroke patients.[99] Nevertheless, the engagement in cognitive, social, and physical activities has been associated with slower cognitive decline in observational studies and was thus thought to increase cognitive reserve.[51,53] Furthermore, stimulating activities may have a positive impact on motivation and may decrease depressive symptoms.

Even though evidence from interventional trials is missing, cognitive activities and mental enrichment even late in life might be a chance to preserve cognition as long as possible. Indeed, a large German population study showed that processing speed improved over a six-year period from 2006 to 2012 when 50–90-year-old persons were tested at the same age.[100] This age-adjusted improvement in cognitive abilities may reflect a cognitively more demanding lifestyle due to modern technology in everyday life and work. Hence, while life expectancy increases, cognitive aging may also be delayed.

Computerized cognitive training is becoming more and more popular. The interest in novel cognitive training platforms, computers, and video games has also increased in the older population, and commercial brain exercises have been developed to improve cognition and delay dementia. In older community-dwelling adults, these training programs were found to improve cognitive abilities and seem to be comparable to traditional paper-and-pencil cognitive training approaches.[101] However, evidence for stroke patients is still lacking. Nevertheless, these interventions are cost effective, flexible, and personalized alternatives to traditional cognitive training programs and may have good adherence because they are designed as games.

Cognitive stimulation, such as a range of enjoyable activities providing general stimulation for thinking, concentration, and memory in a social setting, was found to improve cognitive function and self-reported quality of life in people with mild to moderate dementia.[102]

Furthermore, listening to music was found not only to enhance verbal memory and focused attention at three and six months poststroke but also to induce neuroanatomical changes in the brain.[103,104]

Social Support

High levels of social support and large social networks have been associated with lower mortality risk, lower incidence of cardiovascular disease or stroke, lower risk of cognitive decline or dementia, and an improved recovery after stroke.[105] Furthermore, social support is a protective factor for poststroke depressive symptoms. Observational data suggest that social ties and emotional support at baseline may be associated with a better cognitive outcome at six-months poststroke.[106] However, psychosocial interventions used in this study, and intended to improve social support, did not alter social relationships or increase self-efficacy.

The molecular mechanisms that connect social interventions to cognitive impairment or stroke are yet not fully understood. However, studies suggest that the integrity of the hypothalamic–pituitary–adrenal (HPA) axis, autonomic dysregulation, and changes in systemic inflammation are involved. Social isolation and the feeling of loneliness act as stressors and have been associated with elevated cortisol levels and with heightened inflammation reflected by elevated level of C-reactive protein and by pro-inflammatory cytokineses such as interleukin-6. Elevated cortisol and interleukin-6 levels have been associated with impairment in cognition.[105] Furthermore, decreased levels of brain-derived neurotropic factor (BDNF) were observed as a consequence of social isolation and may play a role in cognitive reserve because BDNF has repeatedly been associated with neuroplasticity.

Social integration and emotional support may thus offer the chance to improve outcome after stroke and to preserve cognition not only in the acute setting but also as a long-term strategy.

References

1. Pendlebury ST, Rothwell PM. Prevalence, incidence, and factors associated with pre-stroke and post-stroke dementia: a systematic review and meta-analysis. *Lancet Neurol.* 2009;8:1006–1018.

2. Hénon H, Pasquier F, Leys D. Poststroke dementia. *Cerebrovasc Dis.* 2006;22:61–70.

3. Godefroy O, Fickl A, Roussel M, et al. Is the Montreal Cognitive Assessment superior to the Mini-Mental State Examination to detect poststroke cognitive impairment? A study with neuropsychological evaluation. *Stroke.* 2011;42:1712–1716.

4. Hurford R, Charidimou A, Fox Z, Cipolotti L, Werring DJ. Domain-specific trends in cognitive impairment after acute ischaemic stroke. *J Neurol.* 2013;**260**:237–241.

5. Leśniak M, Bak T, Czepiel W, Seniów J, Członkowska A. Frequency and prognostic value of cognitive disorders in stroke patients. *Dement Geriatr Cogn Disord.* 2008;**26**:356–363.

6. Nys GMS, van Zandvoort MJE, de Kort PLM, Jansen BPW, de Haan EHF, Kappelle LJ. Cognitive disorders in acute stroke: prevalence and clinical determinants. *Cerebrovasc Dis.* 2007;**23**:408–416.

7. Douiri A, Rudd AG, Wolfe CDA. Prevalence of poststroke cognitive impairment: South London Stroke Register 1995–2010. *Stroke.* 2013;**44**:138–145.

8. Popović IM, Serić V, Demarin V. Mild cognitive impairment in symptomatic and asymptomatic cerebrovascular disease. *J Neurol Sci.* 2007;**257**:185–193.

9. Salvadori E, Pasi M, Poggesi A, Chiti G, Inzitari D, Pantoni L. Predictive value of MoCA in the acute phase of stroke on the diagnosis of mid-term cognitive impairment. *J Neurol.* 2013;**260**:2220–2227.

10. Srikanth VK, Anderson JFI, Donnan GA, et al. Progressive dementia after first-ever stroke: a community-based follow-up study. *Neurology.* 2004;**63**:785–792.

11. Qu Y, Zhuo L, Li N, et al. Prevalence of post-stroke cognitive impairment in China: a community-based, cross-sectional study. *PloS One.* 2015;**10**:e0122864.

12. Demeyere N, Riddoch MJ, Slavkova ED, et al. Domain-specific versus generalized cognitive screening in acute stroke. *J Neurol.* 2016;**263**:306–315.

13. Dacosta-Aguayo R, Graña M, Iturria-Medina Y, et al. Impairment of functional integration of the default mode network correlates with cognitive outcome at three months after stroke. *Hum Brain Mapp.* 2015;**36**:577–590.

14. Zhu Y, Bai L, Liang P, Kang S, Gao H, Yang H. Disrupted brain connectivity networks in acute ischemic stroke patients. *Brain Imaging Behav.* 2017;**11**:444–453.

15. Ballard C, Rowan E, Stephens S, Kalaria R, Kenny RA. Prospective follow-up study between 3 and 15 months after stroke: improvements and decline in cognitive function among dementia-free stroke survivors >75 years of age. *Stroke.* 2003;**34**:2440–2444.

16. Rasquin SMC, Verhey FRJ, Lousberg R, Winkens I, Lodder J. Vascular cognitive disorders: memory, mental speed and cognitive flexibility after stroke. *J Neurol Sci.* 2002;**203**,204:115–119.

17. Rasquin SMC, Lodder J, Verhey FRJ. Predictors of reversible mild cognitive impairment after stroke: a 2-year follow-up study. *J Neurol Sci.* 2005;**229**,230:21–25.

18. Pendlebury ST, Wadling S, Silver LE, Mehta Z, Rothwell PM. Transient cognitive impairment in TIA and minor stroke. *Stroke.* 2011;**42**:3116–3121.

19. Appelros P, Andersson AG. Changes in Mini Mental State Examination score after stroke: lacunar infarction predicts cognitive decline. *Eur J Neurol.* 2006;**13**:491–495.

20. van Zandvoort MJE, Kessels RPC, Nys GMS, de Haan EHF, Kappelle LJ. Early neuropsychological evaluation in patients with ischaemic stroke provides valid information. *Clin Neurol Neurosurg.* 2005;**107**:385–392.

21. Levine DA, Galecki AT, Langa KM, et al. Trajectory of cognitive decline after incident stroke. *JAMA.* 2015;**314**:41–51.

22. Pasquier F, Leys D. Why are stroke patients prone to develop dementia? *J Neurol.* 1997;**244**:135–142.

23. Kalaria RN, Akinyemi R, Ihara M. Stroke injury, cognitive impairment and vascular dementia. *Biochim Biophys Acta.* 2016;**1862**:915–925.

24. Mok VCT, Lam BYK, Wang Z, et al. Delayed-onset dementia after stroke or transient ischemic attack. *Alzheimers Dement.* 2016;**12**:1167–1176.

25. Wang Z, Wong A, Liu W, et al. Cerebral microbleeds and cognitive function in ischemic stroke or transient ischemic attack patients. *Dement Geriatr Cogn Disord.* 2015;**40**:130–136.

26. Arba F, Quinn T, Hankey GJ, et al. Cerebral small vessel disease, medial temporal lobe atrophy and cognitive status in patients with ischaemic stroke and transient ischaemic attack. *Eur J Neurol.* 2017;**24**:276–282.

27. Corraini P, Henderson VW, Ording AG, Pedersen L, Horváth-Puhó E, Sørensen HT. Long-term risk of dementia among survivors of ischemic or hemorrhagic stroke. *Stroke.* 2017;**48**:180–186.

28. Tay SY, Ampil ER, Chen CPLH, Auchus AP. The relationship between homocysteine, cognition and stroke subtypes in acute stroke. *J Neurol Sci.* 2006;**250**:58–61.

29. Munsch F, Sagnier S, Asselineau J, et al. Stroke location is an independent predictor of cognitive outcome. *Stroke.* 2016;**47**:66–73.

30. Lawrence AJ, Brookes RL, Zeestraten EA, Barrick TR, Morris RG, Markus HS. Pattern and rate of cognitive decline in cerebral small vessel disease: a prospective study. *PloS One.* 2015;**10**: e0135523.

31. Makin SDJ, Turpin S, Dennis MS, Wardlaw JM. Cognitive impairment after lacunar stroke: systematic review and meta-analysis of incidence, prevalence and comparison with other stroke subtypes. *J Neurol Neurosurg Psychiatry.* 2013;**84**:893–900.

32. Reijmer YD, Freeze WM, Leemans A, Biessels GJ, Utrecht vascular cognitive impairment study group. The effect of lacunar infarcts on white matter tract integrity. *Stroke.* 2013;**44**:2019–2021.

33. Tang J, Zhong S, Chen Y, et al. Aberrant white matter networks mediate cognitive impairment in patients with silent lacunar infarcts in basal ganglia territory. *J Cereb Blood Flow Metab.* 2015;**35**:1426–1434.

34. Pannese E. Morphological changes in nerve cells during normal aging. *Brain Struct Funct.* 2011;**216**:85–89.

35. Schaapsmeerders P, Maaijwee NAM, van Dijk EJ, et al. Long-term cognitive impairment after first-ever ischemic stroke in young adults. *Stroke.* 2013;**44**:1621–1628.

36. Kivipelto M, Ngandu T, Fratiglioni L, et al. Obesity and vascular risk factors at midlife and the risk of dementia and Alzheimer disease. *Arch Neurol.* 2005;**62**:1556–1560.

37. Beydoun MA, Beydoun HA, Gamaldo AA, Teel A, Zonderman AB, Wang Y. Epidemiologic studies of modifiable factors associated with cognition and dementia: systematic review and meta-analysis. *BMC Public Health.* 2014;**14**:643.

38. Eskelinen MH, Ngandu T, Tuomilehto J, Soininen H, Kivipelto M. Midlife healthy-diet index and late-life dementia and Alzheimer's disease. *Dement Geriatr Cogn Disord Extra.* 2011;**1**:103–112.

39. Kalantarian S, Stern TA, Mansour M, Ruskin JN. Cognitive impairment associated with atrial fibrillation: a meta-analysis. *Ann Intern Med.* 2013;**158**:338–346.

40. Elias MF, Sullivan LM, D'Agostino RB, et al. Framingham Stroke Risk Profile and lowered cognitive performance. *Stroke.* 2004;**35**:404–409.

41. Llewellyn DJ, Lang IA, Xie J, Huppert FA, Melzer D, Langa KM. Framingham Stroke Risk Profile and poor cognitive function: a population-based study. *BMC Neurol.* 2008;**8**:12.

42. Beason-Held LL, Thambisetty M, Deib G, et al. Baseline cardiovascular risk predicts subsequent changes in resting brain function. *Stroke.* 2012;**43**:1542–1547.

43. Lu D, Ren S, Zhang J, Sun D. Vascular risk factors aggravate cognitive impairment in first-ever young ischaemic stroke patients. *Eur J Neurol.* 2016;**23**:940–947.

44. Giau VV, Bagyinszky E, An SSA, Kim SY. Role of apolipoprotein E in neurodegenerative diseases.

Neuropsychiatr Dis Treat. 2015;**11**:1723–1737.

45. Narasimhalu K, Lee J, Leong YL, et al. Inflammatory markers and their association with post stroke cognitive decline. *Int J Stroke.* 2015;**10**:513–518.

46. Kliper E, Bashat DB, Bornstein NM, et al. Cognitive decline after stroke: relation to inflammatory biomarkers and hippocampal volume. *Stroke.* 2013;**44**:1433–1435.

47. Rothenburg LS, Herrmann N, Swardfager W, et al. The relationship between inflammatory markers and post stroke cognitive impairment. *J Geriatr Psychiatry Neurol.* 2010;**23**:199–205.

48. Wang Q, Capistrant BD, Ehntholt A, Glymour MM. Long-term rate of change in memory functioning before and after stroke onset. *Stroke.* 2012;**43**:2561–2566.

49. Rostamian S, Mahinrad S, Stijnen T, Sabayan B, de Craen AJM. Cognitive impairment and risk of stroke: a systematic review and meta-analysis of prospective cohort studies. *Stroke.* 2014;**45**:1342–1348.

50. DeFries T, Avendaño M, Glymour MM. Level and change in cognitive test scores predict risk of first stroke. *J Am Geriatr Soc.* 2009;**57**:499–505.

51. Stern Y. Cognitive reserve in ageing and Alzheimer's disease. *Lancet Neurol.* 2012;**11**:1006–1012.

52. Boyle PA, Wilson RS, Yu L, et al. Much of late life cognitive decline is not due to common neurodegenerative pathologies. *Ann Neurol.* 2013;**74**:478–489.

53. Wang H-X, Jin Y, Hendrie HC, et al. Late life leisure activities and risk of cognitive decline. *J Gerontol A Biol Sci Med Sci.* 2013;**68**:205–213.

54. Nunnari D, Bramanti P, Marino S. Cognitive reserve in stroke and traumatic brain injury patients. *Neurol Sci.* 2014;**35**:1513–1518.

55. Wong A, Lau AYL, Lo E, et al. Relations between recent past leisure activities with risks of dementia and cognitive functions after stroke. *PloS One.* 2016;**11**:e0159952.

56. Alladi S, Bak TH, Mekala S, et al. Impact of bilingualism on cognitive outcome after stroke. *Stroke.* 2016;**47**:258–261.

57. Pendlebury ST, Mariz J, Bull L, Mehta Z, Rothwell PM. MoCA, ACE-R, and MMSE versus the National Institute of Neurological Disorders and Stroke–Canadian Stroke Network Vascular Cognitive Impairment Harmonization Standards Neuropsychological Battery after TIA and stroke. *Stroke.* 2012;**43**:464–469.

58. Srikanth VK, Quinn SJ, Donnan GA, Saling MM, Thrift AG. Long-term cognitive transitions, rates of cognitive change, and predictors of incident dementia in a population-based first-ever stroke cohort. *Stroke J Cereb Circ.* 2006;**37**:2479–2483.

59. Hachinski V, Iadecola C, Petersen RC, et al. National Institute of Neurological Disorders and Stroke⁻Canadian Stroke Network vascular cognitive impairment harmonization standards. *Stroke.* 2006;**37**:2220–2241.

60. Maruta C, Guerreiro M, de Mendonça A, Hort J, Scheltens P. The use of neuropsychological tests across Europe: the need for a consensus in the use of assessment tools for dementia. *Eur J Neurol.* 2011;**18**:279–285.

61. Eskes GA, Lanctôt KL, Herrmann N, et al. Canadian Stroke Best Practice Recommendations: Mood, Cognition and Fatigue Following Stroke practice guidelines, update 2015. *Int J Stroke.* 2015;**10**:1130–1140.

62. Lees R, Selvarajah J, Fenton C, et al. Test accuracy of cognitive screening tests for diagnosis of dementia and multidomain cognitive impairment in stroke. *Stroke.* 2014;**45**:3008–3018.

63. van Rijsbergen MWA, Mark RE, de Kort PLM, Sitskoorn MM. Subjective cognitive complaints after stroke: a systematic review. *J Stroke Cerebrovasc Dis.* 2014;**23**:408–420.

64. van Rijsbergen MWA, Mark RE, Kop WJ, de Kort PLM, Sitskoorn MM. The role of objective cognitive dysfunction in

subjective cognitive complaints after stroke. *Eur J Neurol.* 2017;**24**:475–482.

65. Harrison JK, Fearon P, Noel-Storr AH, McShane R, Stott DJ, Quinn TJ. Informant Questionnaire on Cognitive Decline in the Elderly (IQCODE) for the diagnosis of dementia within a secondary care setting. *Cochrane Database Syst Rev.* 2015;**3**: CD010772.

66. Leys D, Hénon H, Mackowiak-Cordoliani M-A, Pasquier F. Poststroke dementia. *Lancet Neurol.* 2005;**4**:752–759.

67. Grysiewicz R, Gorelick PB. Key neuroanatomical structures for post-stroke cognitive impairment. *Curr Neurol Neurosci Rep.* 2012;**12**:703–708.

68. Kliper E, Ben Assayag E, Tarrasch R, et al. Cognitive state following stroke: the predominant role of preexisting white matter lesions. *PloS One.* 2014;**9**:e105461.

69. Kooistra M, Geerlings MI, van der Graaf Y, et al. Vascular brain lesions, brain atrophy, and cognitive decline: The Second Manifestations of ARTerial disease–Magnetic Resonance (SMART-MR) study. *Neurobiol Aging.* 2014;**35**:35–41.

70. Brainin M, Tuomilehto J, Heiss W-D, et al. Post-stroke cognitive decline: an update and perspectives for clinical research. *Eur J Neurol.* 2015;**22**:229–238, e13–16.

71. Dichgans M, Zietemann V. Prevention of vascular cognitive impairment. *Stroke.* 2012;**43**:3137–3146.

72. Cicerone KD, Langenbahn DM, Braden C, et al. Evidence-based cognitive rehabilitation: updated review of the literature from 2003 through 2008. *Arch Phys Med Rehabil.* 2011;**92**:519–530.

73. Rohling ML, Faust ME, Beverly B, Demakis G. Effectiveness of cognitive rehabilitation following acquired brain injury: a meta-analytic re-examination of Cicerone et al.'s (2000, 2005) systematic reviews. *Neuropsychology.* 2009;**23**: 20–39.

74. das Nair R, Cogger H, Worthington E, Lincoln NB. Cognitive rehabilitation for memory deficits after stroke. *Cochrane Database Syst Rev.* 2016;**9**:CD002293.

75. Loetscher T, Lincoln NB. Cognitive rehabilitation for attention deficits following stroke. *Cochrane Database Syst Rev.* 2013;**5**:CD002842.

76. Chung CSY, Pollock A, Campbell T, Durward BR, Hagen S. Cognitive rehabilitation for executive dysfunction in adults with stroke or other adult non-progressive acquired brain damage. *Cochrane Database Syst Rev.* 2013;**4**: CD008391.

77. Bath PM, Wardlaw JM. Pharmacological treatment and prevention of cerebral small vessel disease: a review of potential interventions. *Int J Stroke.* 2015;**10**:469–478.

78. Hackett ML, Pickles K. Part I: frequency of depression after stroke: an updated systematic review and meta-analysis of observational studies. *Int J Stroke.* 2014;**9**:1017–1025.

79. Hackett ML, Anderson CS, House A, Xia J. Interventions for treating depression after stroke. *Cochrane Database Syst Rev.* 2008;**4**: CD003437.

80. Mead GE, Hsieh C-F, Lee R, et al. Selective serotonin reuptake inhibitors (SSRIs) for stroke recovery. *Cochrane Database Syst Rev.* 2012;**11**:CD009286.

81. Ngandu T, Lehtisalo J, Solomon A, et al. A 2 year multidomain intervention of diet, exercise, cognitive training, and vascular risk monitoring versus control to prevent cognitive decline in at-risk elderly people (FINGER): a randomised controlled trial. *Lancet.* 2015;**385**:2255–2263.

82. Moll van Charante EP, Richard E, Eurelings LS, et al. Effectiveness of a 6-year multidomain vascular care intervention to prevent dementia (preDIVA): a cluster-randomised controlled trial. *Lancet.* 2016;**388**:797–805.

83. Matz K, Teuschl Y, Firlinger B, et al. Multidomain lifestyle interventions for the prevention of cognitive decline after ischemic stroke: randomized trial. *Stroke.* 2015;**46**:2874–2880.

84. Ihle-Hansen H, Thommessen B, Fagerland MW, et al. Multifactorial vascular risk factor intervention to prevent

cognitive impairment after stroke and TIA: a 12-month randomized controlled trial. *Int J Stroke.* 2014;**9**:932–938.

85. Ihle-Hansen H, Thommessen B, Fagerland MW, et al. Effect on anxiety and depression of a multifactorial risk factor intervention program after stroke and TIA: a randomized controlled trial. *Aging Ment Health.* 2014;**18**:540–546.

86. Douiri A, McKevitt C, Emmett ES, Rudd AG, Wolfe CDA. Long-term effects of secondary prevention on cognitive function in stroke patients. *Circulation.* 2013;**128**:1341–1348.

87. Bath PM, Scutt P, Blackburn DJ, et al. Intensive versus guideline blood pressure and lipid lowering in patients with previous stroke: main results from the Pilot "Prevention of Decline in Cognition after Stroke Trial" (PODCAST) randomised controlled trial. *PloS One.* 2017;**12**: e0164608.

88. Valls-Pedret C, Sala-Vila A, Serra-Mir M, et al. Mediterranean diet and age-related cognitive decline: a randomized clinical trial. *JAMA Intern Med.* 2015;**175**:1094–1103.

89. Ursin MH, Bergland A, Fure B, Tørstad A, Tveit A, Ihle-Hansen H. Balance and mobility as predictors of post-stroke cognitive impairment. *Dement Geriatr Cogn Disord Extra.* 2015;**5**:203–211.

90. Constans A, Pin-Barre C, Temprado J-J, Decherchi P, Laurin J. Influence of aerobic training and combinations of interventions on cognition and neuroplasticity after stroke. *Front Aging Neurosci.* 2016;**8**:164.

91. Tiozzo E, Youbi M, Dave K, et al. Aerobic, resistance, and cognitive exercise training poststroke. *Stroke.* 2015;**46**:2012–2016.

92. Jones F, Riazi A. Self-efficacy and self-management after stroke: a systematic review. *Disabil Rehabil.* 2011;**33**:797–810.

93. Visser MM, Aben L, Heijenbrok-Kal MH, Busschbach JJV, Ribbers GM. The relative effect of coping strategy and depression on health-related quality of life in patients in the chronic phase after stroke. *J Rehabil Med.* 2014;**46**:514–519.

94. Marzolini S, Balitsky A, Jagroop D, et al. Factors affecting attendance at an adapted cardiac rehabilitation exercise program for individuals with mobility deficits poststroke. *J Stroke Cerebrovasc Dis.* Epub. 2015 Sep. 28.

95. Banks G, Bernhardt J, Churilov L, Cumming TB. Exercise preferences are different after stroke. *Stroke Res Treat.* 2012;**2012**:890946.

96. Prout EC, Brooks D, Mansfield A, Bayley M, McIlroy WE. Patient characteristics that influence enrollment and attendance in aerobic exercise early after stroke. *Arch Phys Med Rehabil.* 2015;**96**:823–830.

97. Pfaeffli Dale L, Dobson R, Whittaker R, Maddison R. The effectiveness of mobile-health behaviour change interventions for cardiovascular disease self-management: a systematic review. *Eur J Prev Cardiol.* 2016; **23**:801-817.

98. Pal K, Eastwood SV, Michie S, et al. Computer-based diabetes self-management interventions for adults with type 2 diabetes mellitus. *Cochrane Database Syst Rev.* 2013;**3**:CD008776.

99. Corbett D, Nguemeni C, Gomez-Smith M. How can you mend a broken brain? Neurorestorative approaches to stroke recovery. *Cerebrovasc Dis.* 2014;**38**:233–239.

100. Steiber N. Population aging at cross-roads: diverging secular trends in average cognitive functioning and physical health in the older population of Germany. *PloS One.* 2015;**10**:e0136583.

101. Kueider AM, Parisi JM, Gross AL, Rebok GW. Computerized cognitive training with older adults: a systematic review. *PloS One.* 2012;**7**:e40588.

102. Woods B, Aguirre E, Spector AE, Orrell M. Cognitive stimulation to improve cognitive functioning in people with dementia. *Cochrane Database Syst Rev.* 2012;**2**:CD005562.

103. Särkämö T, Tervaniemi M, Laitinen S, et al. Music listening enhances cognitive recovery and mood after middle cerebral

artery stroke. *Brain J Neurol.* 2008;**131**:866–876.

104. Särkämö T, Ripollés P, Vepsäläinen H, et al. Structural changes induced by daily music listening in the recovering brain after middle cerebral artery stroke: a voxel-based morphometry study. *Front Hum Neurosci.* 2014;**8**:245.

105. Friedler B, Crapser J, McCullough L. One is the deadliest number: the detrimental effects of social isolation on cerebrovascular diseases and cognition. *Acta Neuropathol.* 2015;**129**:493–509.

106. Glymour MM, Weuve J, Fay ME, Glass T, Berkman LF. Social ties and cognitive recovery after stroke: does social integration promote cognitive resilience? *Neuroepidemiology.* 2008;**31**:10–20.

Reversible Dementias

Lawrence S. Honig

Introduction

Dementia is defined as a change in cognition and/or behavior affecting function of the individual[1] By definition, dementia must be a change or progression from the prior state of "normality." At the current time, the most common dementias are indeed irreversible. These involve age-related neurodegeneration, or of damage to the brain by trauma or vascular insults. These dementia disorders have treatments, but no proven disease modifying therapies. Extensive research is being performed to develop therapies to slow the course, stabilize, or reverse the deficits of these disorders, but currently the only treatments are symptomatic.[2,3] Such treatments do not slow or reverse the dementia process, but ameliorate symptoms and palliate, and include antidepressants, anxiolytics, anticonvulsants, antipsychotics, and other symptomatic drugs as well as the cholinesterase inhibitors to improve symptoms in Alzheimer's and Lewy body dementia processes. While there are no disease modifying or reversing treatments for the more common dementias, there are an important spectrum of dementia conditions that owe to neoplastic, toxic, metabolic, inflammatory, infectious, or hydrocephalic causes, many of which are potentially reversible. In some cases, even a neurodegenerative condition, may be accompanied by an additional component of one of these "reversible dementia" conditions. These "reversible" dementias are the subject of this chapter.

Neoplastic Dementias

Before twentieth century imaging, dementia due to unrecognized brain neoplasm was more common. Now that neuroimaging by computerized tomography (CT) or magnetic resonance imaging (MRI) has achieved such wide penetration into clinical practice, uncovering the presence of brain lesions responsible for dementia is usually quite prompt. Typically a subacute change in mentation affecting daily functioning, but not obviously due to a focal process, is due to a diffuse white matter, frontal, or right hemispheric process.[4] Meningiomas with edema, and astrocytomas (typically glioblastomas) are most common, since the progressive edema and mass effect causes mental dysfunction. The dementia caused by these lesions, is typically temporized by steroids, and relieved by surgery and/or radiotherapy, with increasing use of chemotherapy. Another class of dementias caused by neoplasms are the "paraneoplastic" dementias, which involve brain dysfunction due to an autoimmune mechanism, triggered typically by a peripheral (non-nervous system) tumor. Many of these dementias can be reversed, but they are discussed later in this chapter under inflammatory dementias.

Table 7.1 Reversible toxic dementias

	Exposure source	Common concomitant features
Heavy Metals		
Lead	Lead-acid batteries	Gastrointestinal symptoms, neuropathy
Mercury	Mining	Psychosis, neuropathy
Arsenic	Insecticides/rodenticides	Neuropathy, abdominal pain
Manganese	Manufacturing	Neuropathy
Volatile substances		
Toluene	Airplane glue	Impaired consciousness

Toxic Dementias

In the developed world, toxic causes of dementia are uncommon.[5] Exposures to heavy metals and volatile organics are historical causes of dementia. These dementia conditions may reverse with removal of the source of exposure, and subsequent clearance from the body of the toxic substance, whether by passage of time, or through the aid of therapeutic moieties. See Table 7.1 for a list of such toxic agents. Heavy metal toxicity causing dementia, whether from lead, mercury, manganese, arsenic, or other elements is now extremely rare in North America.[5] Lead poisoning has occurred in less developed areas, mostly due to processing of lead-acid batteries without adequate protection. Arsenic poisoning may occur from intentional criminal poisoning. Toxic dementia due to inhalation of volatile organics, is an ongoing problem, particularly in younger persons due to recreational use of volatile substances, such as 'glue sniffing' to become "high."[6] Another uncommon cause of dementia is chronic exposure to carbon monoxide.[7] Discontinuation of the toxic exposure may lead to partial or complete reversal of the dementia. For heavy metal poisoning, chelation therapy can lead to more prompt recovery.

Metabolic Dementias

Metabolic causes of dementia are uncommon, but include vitamin deficiencies, hypothyroidism, hypoadrenalism, hyperparathyroidism, uremia, hepatic failure, porphyria, and other rarer conditions. Vitamin deficiencies include Vitamin B12 (cyanocobalamin), vitamin B1 (thiamine) deficiency, niacin deficiency, and rarer deficiencies.[8] See Table 7.2 for a list of metabolic causes of dementia, the only somewhat common vitamin deficiency in North America is B12 deficiency, which is sometimes a nutritional deficiency, but typically occurs from inability of gastric mucosa to uptake the vitamin, otherwise known as cyanocobalamin. This incapacity may result from prior surgical resections, or more commonly from autoimmune destruction of the important gastric parietal cells. Symptoms may be subacute over months, or chronic over years, and include diffuse cognitive dysfunction,[9] sometimes psychotic symptoms, and almost universally demyelinating dorsal column deficits causing proprioceptive loss, and small-fiber peripheral neuropathy. Diagnosis can be made on the basis of low B12 levels in serum. However, without confirmatory testing

Table 7.2 Reversible metabolic dementias

	Common etiology	Common concomitant features
Vitamin Disorders		
Vitamin B12 deficiency	GI surgery, autoimmune	Neuropathy, psychosis
Niacin deficiency	Nutritional	Diarrhea, neuropathy
Thiamine deficiency	Alcoholism	Oculomotor paresis, nystagmus, ataxia
Endocrine Disorders		
Hypothyroidism	Autoimmune, postsurgical	Weight gain, bradycardia, skin changes
Hypoadrenalism	Autoimmune, postsurgical	Lethargy
Medical Disorders		
Uremia	Renal failure or obstruction	Somnolence, pruritis, restless legs, asterixis
Hepatic Failure	Hepatitis, cirrhosis, biliary	Confusion, somnolence, asterixis

showing elevation of both serum methylmalonate and homocysteine, it is unlikely that the low B12 levels are functionally important and related to cognitive change. Once B12 deficiency is confirmed, it is useful to measure anti-parietal cell antibody, to establish whether gastric mucosa, assuming it is surgically undisturbed, is functioning, in which case oral supplementation with B12 may be sufficient to reverse the deficiency, or to establish that parietal cell antibodies are present, in which case it is wise to supplement B12, initially through weekly, then through monthly intramuscular injections. Thiamine deficiency (vitamin B1) typically causes a subacute or acute dementia known as Wernicke-Korsakoff's syndrome.[10] The dominant characteristic is memory dysfunction and confabulation, and results from necrotic changes in the mammillary bodies and thalami, which sometimes can now be imaged using MRI. Common clinical accompaniments are paresis of extraocular movements, nystagmus, and ataxia. The setting of vitamin B1 deficiency is typically alcoholism. Dementia can be stabilized and partially reversed by prompt treatment with thiamine, preferably given intravenously. Laboratory blood tests have not been proven useful, although there may be some possibly utility of thiamine levels and red cell transketolase activity measurements. Regardless, treatment should be initiated, immediately after blood draw, and should not await return of results. Hypothyroidism is nowadays a rare cause of subacute or chronic dementia, with mental slowing and apathy being the dominant features.[11,12] The dysfunction usually results from autoimmune thyroid destruction (Hashimoto's disease, or thyroidectomies, without adequate postsurgical hormone replacement). Medical concomitant features of weight gain, bradycardia, hyperlipidemia, pretibial edema, and other skin and hair changes may be present in marked cases. Treatment with thyroxine supplementation typically results in reversal of symptoms. Hyperparathyroidism causes subacute dementia through hypercalcemia. It commonly presents with confusion and psychiatric symptoms. Kidney failure (uremia) and hepatic failure both cause subacute or chronic dementias with confusion, mental fluctuations, psychiatric symptoms, and motor findings including asterixis and myoclonus.

Neuroinfectious Dementias

Infectious causes of dementia are more common than toxic or metabolic, but still relatively uncommon in North America. Table 7.3 lists a variety of infections that cause progressive dementia, usually subacute, and are all treatable to a lesser or greater degree. Viral meningitides, including herpes simplex encephalitis, may have some reversibility with antiviral treatment, and HIV encephalitis[13] may improve with antiretroviral therapy. Lyme disease may cause a subacute or chronic encephalopathy, but it is very uncommon as a dementia cause. Likewise, syphilis, in earlier centuries not such an uncommon cause, is now rare.[14,15] Both of the spirochetal disorders may be diagnosed when there is inflammatory cerebrospinal fluid (CSF), with antibody evidence of CNS involvement, or PCR evidence of organismal genome in the CSF. Atypical mycobacterium, such as tuberculosis, usually causes a more subacute dementia, and typically systemic involvement may be evident, but again is diagnosed by cellular CSF and positive assays for tubercular organisms, proteins, or genome. Cryptococcal meningitis, coccidial meningitis, and less commonly histoplasmal meningitis are all fungal causes of subacute or chronic dementia.[16] Like the other infectious dementias, the clinical syndrome is usually of more subacute course, diffuse cerebral

Table 7.3 Reversible neuroinfectious dementias

	Exposure source	Common concomitant features
Viral		
Herpes simplex	Person-to-person /reactivation	Genital or oral ulcer history
Herpes zoster	Prior chickenpox/reactivation	Skin vesicles over a dermatome
Spirochetal		
Lyme	Tick-borne	Prior rash, arthritis, carditis
Syphilis	Sexual transmission	Prior genital disease, arthritis, aortitis
Atypical bacterial		
Tuberculosis	Respiratory person-to-person	Pulmonary disease
Fungal		
Cryptococcus	Immunosuppression	Fevers, stiff neck, gait disorder
Coccidiomycosis	Soil, California Central Valley	Fevers, stiff neck, gait disorder
Histoplasmosis	caves, bats, birds	
Parasitic		
Cysticercosis	Fecal oral contamination	Various focal neurological symptoms
Toxoplasmosis	Cat feces	Various focal neurological symptoms

involvement, and the hallmarks are CSF inflammation and presence of organisms by antigen-testing, PCR testing, or high antibody index, indicating CNS involvement. Cerebral cysticercosis and toxoplasmosis are organismal parasitoses that are usually evident on neuroimaging due to formation of discrete lesions or abscesses, and confirmed by antibody testing and/or biopsy in some cases.

The nonviral infectious causes of dementia may be quite treatable, with stabilization, or considerable reversal of symptoms. Lyme and syphilis can be treated with cephalosporins or penicillins.[14] Tuberculosis can be treated with tuberculocidal therapies, including isoniazid, rifampin, pyrazinamide, and streptomycin. Fungal meningitides can often be treated with antifungal drugs such as fluconazole, itraconazole, as well as amphotericin. Cysticercosis can be treated with praziquantel, or albendazole. Toxoplasmosis is treated by pyrimethamine-sulfisoxazole.

Not all infectious causes of dementia are treatable. Subacute sclerosing panencephalitis is a smoldering viral disease due to measles or mumps, with no clear treatment. Other viral encephalitic disorders causing dementia such as rabies or progressive multifocal leukoencephalopathy (PML) also have no effective treatments. Likewise certain fungal disorders, such as blastomycosis, and parasitic disorders such as Naeglarial (amoebic) encephalitis are rarely reversed.

Inflammatory Dementia Disorders

Inflammatory causes of dementia, are the most common causes of subacute, reversible dementia. These include CNS involvement from systemic inflammatory disorders, such as systemic lupus erythematosus, specific demyelinating CNS disorders, including multiple sclerosis, and its variants, and a number of recently recognized specifically neuroinflammatory disorders characterized by the presence of specific neuronal autoantibodies. Some of these disorders are delineated in Table 7.4.

Systemic Inflammatory Disorders

Disorders such as systemic lupus, sarcoidosis, Wegener's granulomatosis, and others, are systemic inflammatory disorders that may present isolated to the central nervous system, or with predominant CNS involvement. These disorders, when present in the brain, causing progressive dementia, are usually subacute, and usually respond with stabilization and partial or full reversal of dementia upon administration of immune therapies, delivered in similar fashion to those delivered for their systemic versions. The primary modalities for therapy are glucocorticosteroids and intravenous immunoglobulin G. In some of the antibody-mediated disorders, plasmapheresis is used, particularly in catastrophic cases. In cases of disease that is refractory to primary modalities, or in cases of relapses with reductions of steroids, appropriate therapies include graduation to more potent treatments including ablation of B-cell lymphocytes with rituximab, or more general immunosuppression with azathioprine, mycophenolate, or cyclophosphamide as required.

CNS Demyelinating Disorders

Multiple sclerosis, and its variants including sometimes neuromyelitis optica, may present as primary dementias,[17] but usually motoric, sensory, and cerebellar features are evident.

Table 7.4 Reversible neuroinflammatory dementias

	Exposure source	Common concomitant features
"Systemic" disorders		
Systemic lupus	Unknown, genetic?	Arthritis, blood, renal, skin disease
Sarcoidosis	Unknown, genetic?	Lung disease
Wegener's granulomatosis	Unknown, genetic?	Sinus, lung, renal disease
Demyelinating disorders		
Multiple sclerosis	Unknown, genetic?	Motor, sensory, cerebellar symptoms
Neuromyelitis optica	Unknown, genetic?	Optic nerve, spinal symptoms
Autoimmune disorders		
VGKC complex antibodies	Unknown, paraneoplastic	Seizures, hyponatremia
NMDA-receptor antibody	Unknown, paraneoplastic	Seizures, dyskinesias, psychosis
AMPA-receptor antibody	Unknown	Seizures
mGluR5 antibody	Unknown, lymphoma	Cerebellar ataxia
GABA-A receptor antibody	Unknown	Seizures
GABA-B receptor antibody	Unknown, paraneoplastic	Seizures, ataxia, opsoclonus-myoclonus
GAD65 antibody	Unknown, paraneoplastic	Seizures, pain, stiffness
Glycine-receptor antibody	Unknown, paraneoplastic	Myelitis, rigidity, myoclonus
DPPX-antibody	Unknown, paraneoplastic	Diarrhea, rigidity, ataxia, hyperekplexia
IgLON antibody	Unknown, paraneoplastic	Sleep disorders, autonomic dysfunction
Antithyroid antibodies	Unknown	Headaches, seizures

Abbreviations: VGKC (voltage-gated potassium channel – includes LGI1, leucine-rich glioma-inactivated protein 1, CASPR2, contactin-associated protein-like 2 antibodies); NMDA (N-methyl-D-aspartate); AMPA (α-amino-3-hydroxy-5-methyl-4-isoxazole propionic acid); mGluR5 (metabotropic glutamate receptor 5); GABA (gamma-aminobutyric acid); GAD65 (glutamate acid decarboxylase 65 kilodalton isoform); DPPX (dipeptidyl-peptidase-like protein-6)

Treatment of these demyelinating disorders may result in partial or sometimes complete reversal of dementia syndromes. There are currently a large number of immune-based treatments for demyelinating disease. These treatments typically stabilize disease symptoms, but reversibility of dementia symptoms is usually only partial.

Antibody-Associated Disorders

In the latter part of the twentieth century, it became apparent that subacute dementia may be due to "autoimmune" central nervous system disorders, disorders associated with the presence of syndrome-specific measurable plasma or cerebrospinal fluid antibodies.[18] These disorders can be broadly grouped into disorders marked by antineuronal nuclear antibodies, antineuronal cell surface antibodies, and antibodies of unclear or plural subcellular localizations. Each antibody-associated disorder may have a generally archetypical symptom complex, but presentations and exact features may vary. Many of these disorders are characterized by the presence of headaches or seizures, and some involve motor or cerebellar systems more than dementia, but most are marked by a subacute dementia. Each of these disorders may present as a "pure autoimmune" disorder, in that there is no known cause of the antibody and associated syndrome, or may present as a "paraneoplastic" disorder, in which the presence of a bodily tumor (often very small and otherwise asymptomatic) apparently has provoked the presence of the anti-nervous system antibodies.[19] A special case of "antibody-associated disorders" is called "Hashimoto's encephalitis,"[20] also known as "steroid-responsive encephalitis." As apparent from the names, this is a steroid-responsive subacute dementia, marked by presence of serum antithyroid antibodies – specifically anti-thyroglobulin, anti-thyroperoxidase, and anti-microsomal antibodies.

The reversible disorders are associated with anti-cell-surface antibodies. The disorders associated with antinuclear neuronal antibodies, such as anti-Hu and anti-Yo, have been refractory to treatments – at best stabilization can be achieved when an inciting tumor is removed or treated, but reversal of dementia symptoms has not been achieved. It seems that the reason why the disorders associated with cell-surface antibodies are more reversible, is because the antibodies generally cause neuronal dysfunction due to disturbance of cell receptors, may cause some associated inflammation, but generally do not cause neuronal destruction. The reason why the disorders associated with antinuclear antibodies are irreversible seems to relate to the marked neuronal destruction that occurs in these disorders, typically in the limbic system and brainstem in anti-Hu, and in the cerebellum in anti-Yo syndrome. Evidence is also better that the anti-cell-surface antigen antibodies are actually pathoetiologically responsible for symptoms, while the antinuclear antibodies, may possibly be markers of the disorder rather than disease-causing in and of themselves.

The two most common dementias due to cell-surface antibodies are anti-NMDA receptor antibody encephalitis (NMDARE),[21] and anti-voltage-gated potassium channel (VGKC) complex encephalopathy.[22] NMDARE typically presents subacutely in young adults, usually female (or in the pediatric population) under the age of 45. It is marked by seizures, psychosis, oral-facial-mandibular dystonia and dyskinesias, coma, and autonomic dysfunction (tachycardia, bradycardia, asystole, hyperpyrexia, diaphoresis). It is diagnosed by ascertainment of the presence of NMDA receptor antibody in CSF (also often present in blood), and often is accompanied by inflammatory CSF changes and brain lesions. In about half of cases, the disorder is associated with an ovarian teratoma. Treatment requires tumor removal (if tumor is present), and immune therapies, with steroids, intravenous immunoglobulin, sometimes plasmapheresis, and sometimes rituximab, or more potent immunosuppressants. VGKC complex antibody encephalopathy may also be subacute, or even more chronic, but typically occurs in the elderly, and is marked by memory and cognitive changes, and in most cases by electrographically-negative seizure-like events of brief paroxysmal face and/or arm movements ("facio-brachial seizures"), often lasting only 1 or a few seconds. This disorder can be diagnosed through blood test for the antibody. The LGI1 antibody and CASPR-2 antibody are both members of the VGKC complex family. LGI1 is more associated with facio-brachial seizures. Like NMDA antibody, it is occasionally tumor-associated (typically lung tumors, but less than 10 percent of cases), and is treated similarly with immunomodulatory therapies. However, for this disorder, typically steroids are a mainstay of therapy, and very effective, along with anticonvulsants such as phenytoin.

Hydrocephalic Dementia

Hydrocephalus is defined as increased fluid in the cranial compartment causing compression of brain tissue and consequent central nervous system dysfunction. The classical triad of hydrocephalus is gait disorder, urinary dyscontrol, and dementia.[23] Typically gait disorder and urinary dysfunction may precede significant dementia, but this is not always the case. Gait disorder may be attributed to neuropathy, spinal disease, or arthritic disease, particularly in the elderly. Urinary dysfunction may be attributed to prostatic or other urinary tract issues. Thus, dementia may be the recognized CNS symptom. Typically, the dementia and other symptoms are slowly progressive over some years, although more subacute presentations do occur. There may be fluctuations,which may increase diagnostic uncertainty. Since ventricular enlargement is common, "hydrocephalus" is frequently noted on CT and MRI scans, even if the ventricular enlargement is due to atrophy, and not pathoetiologically contributory to symptoms. There are various imaging features that prompt suspicion of clinically relevant and thus potentially reversible hydrocephalus. These include prominence of ventricles disproportionate to increased sulcal size (suggestive of gyral compression), rounded "ballooned" appearance of ventricles, particularly anteriorly, thinning and bowing of the corpus callosum, and evidence of diffuse-contiguous periventricular white matter T2 signal change (suggestive of transependymal fluid flow).[24]

Historical and examination features that are supportive of hydrocephalus as a cause of dementia include history of meningitis or subarachnoid hemorrhage of any cause at any time in the past (e.g., head trauma or aneurysmal bleeding), and history of typical gait (wide-based, magnetic, "freezing" gait, with postural instability), and urinary (frequency and/or incontinence, not attributable to urological system) symptoms.

Suggestive clinical history, examination, and neuroimaging features are still often insufficient for reasonably certain diagnosis of the presence of reversible dementia due to hydrocephalus. It is likely that in many cases there is "compensated" hydrocephalus, which is noncontributory, and therefore not susceptible to relief of fluid dynamics yielding dementia reversal. For this reason, the hydrocephalus evaluation usually includes a large volume lumbar puncture, preferably with videotaped gait examination before and during the subsequent hours afterwards. Improvement in gait and urination post-removal of CSF volumes of 35 to 50 cc, is suggestive of potential reversibility of dementia. Lumbar puncture also allows analysis of CSF to eliminate possible inflammatory or infectious etiologies. Alternatives to a single large volume lumbar puncture, are several consecutive daily lumbar punctures, or a lumbar drainage procedure, in which an indwelling spinal catheter is placed, allowing fluid removal (e.g. 40 cc every 4 hours) for 3 to 5 days. This latter procedure has the potential for greater chance of observing improvement from CSF diversion, but also can be discomfiting for patients, and has risk of meningitis infection, particularly in more impaired patients, less aware of the presence of the catheter. Once a decision has been made that hydrocephalus may be a contributing etiology to the dementia, then the neurosurgical placement of a ventriculoperitoneal, or ventriculoatrial (particularly in more obese patients) shunt may provide some reversal of dementia symptoms, although in many cases there may be concomitant neurodegeneration.[25,26]

References

1. Cummings JL. Dementia: the failing brain. *Lancet* 1995. **345**: 1481–4.

2. Honig LS. Translational research in neurology: dementia. *Arch Neurol* 2012. **69**: 969–77.

3. Honig LS and Boyd CD. Treatment of Alzheimer's Disease: Current Management and Experimental Therapeutics. *Curr Transl Geriatr Exp Gerontol Rep* 2013. **2**: 174–181.

4. Noble JM, Canoll P, and Honig LS. Brain tumor-associated dementia. *Sci Aging Knowledge Environ* **2005**. 2005: dn2.

5. Schofield P. Dementia associated with toxic causes and autoimmune disease. *Int Psychogeriatr* 2005. **17** Suppl 1: S129–47.

6. Filley CM, Heaton RK, and Rosenberg NL. White matter dementia in chronic toluene abuse. *Neurology* 1990. **40**: 532–4.

7. Lai CY, Huang YW, Tseng CH, et al. Patients With Carbon Monoxide Poisoning and Subsequent Dementia: A Population-Based Cohort Study. *Medicine (Baltimore)* 2016. **95**: e2418.

8. Crystal HA, Ortof E, Frishman WH, et al. Serum vitamin B12 levels and incidence of dementia in a healthy elderly population: a report from the Bronx Longitudinal Aging Study. *J Am Geriatr Soc* 1994. **42**: 933–6.

9. Moore E, Mander A, Ames D, et al. Cognitive impairment and vitamin B12: a review. *Int Psychogeriatr* 2012. **24**: 541–56.

10. Sher L. Wernicke-Korsakoff syndrome and alcohol-induced persistent dementia. *Aust N Z J Psychiatry* 2004. **38**: 976–7.

11. Clarnette RM and Patterson CJ. Hypothyroidism: does treatment cure dementia? *J Geriatr Psychiatry Neurol* 1994. 7: 23–7.

12. Haupt M and Kurz A. Reversibility of dementia in hypothyroidism. *J Neurol* 1993. **240**: 333–5.

13. Nath A, Schiess N, Venkatesan A, et al. Evolution of HIV dementia with HIV infection. *Int Rev Psychiatry* 2008. **20**: 25–31.

14. Nitrini R. Clinical and therapeutic aspects of dementia in syphilis and Lyme disease. *Handb Clin Neurol* 2008. **89**: 819–23.

15. Miklossy J. Biology and neuropathology of dementia in syphilis and Lyme disease. *Handb Clin Neurol* 2008. **89**: 825–44.

16. Gottfredsson M and Perfect JR. Fungal meningitis. *Semin Neurol* 2000. **20**: 307–22.

17. Westervelt HJ. Dementia in multiple sclerosis: why is it rarely discussed? *Arch Clin Neuropsychol* 2015. **30**: 174–7.

18. Dalmau J. NMDA receptor encephalitis and other antibody-mediated disorders of the synapse: The 2016 Cotzias Lecture. *Neurology* 2016. **87**: 2471-82.

19. Graus F, Titulaer MJ, Balu R, et al. A clinical approach to diagnosis of autoimmune encephalitis. *Lancet Neurol* 2016. **15**: 391–404.

20. Laurent C, Capron J, Quillerou B, et al. Steroid-responsive encephalopathy associated with autoimmune thyroiditis (SREAT): characteristics, treatment and outcome in 251 cases from the literature. *Autoimmun Rev* 2016. **15**: 1129–1133.

21. Maccaferri GE, Rossetti AO, Dalmau J, et al. Anti-N-Methyl-D-Aspartate Receptor Encephalitis: A New Challenging Entity for Consultation-Liaison Psychiatrist. *Brain Disord Ther* 2016. **5**.

22. van Sonderen A, Petit-Pedrol M, Dalmau J, Titulaer MJ.The value of LGI1, Caspr2 and voltage-gated potassium channel antibodies in encephalitis. *Nat Rev Neurol* 2017. **13**: 290-301.

23. Williams MA, Malm J. Diagnosis and Treatment of Idiopathic Normal Pressure Hydrocephalus. *Continuum (Minneap Minn)* 2016. **22**: 579–99.

24. Bradley WG, Jr. Magnetic Resonance Imaging of Normal Pressure Hydrocephalus. *Semin Ultrasound CT MR* 2016. **37**: 120–8.

25. Halperin JJ, Kurlan R, Schwalb JM, et al. Practice guideline: Idiopathic normal pressure hydrocephalus: Response to shunting and predictors of response: Report of the Guideline Development, Dissemination, and Implementation Subcommittee of the American Academy of Neurology. *Neurology* 2015. **85**: 2063-71.

26. Espay AJ, Da Prat GA, Dwivedi AK, et al. Deconstructing normal pressure hydrocephalus: ventriculomegaly as early sign of neurodegeneration. *Ann Neurol* 2017. **82**: 503–13.

Chapter 8

Prevention of Dementia

J. David Spence

Introduction

Dementia increases steeply with age. A population-based study in Saskatchewan, Canada, from administrative databases over the period 2001 to 2013, found that the incidence of dementia increased by 2.8 to 5.1 times, and the prevalence increased by 2.6 to 4.6 times, for every 10 years after 45 years of age.[1] With the aging of the population in developed countries, a great increase in the prevalence of dementia is anticipated, resulting in calls for integrated approaches to prevention.[2] However, several recent studies indicate that in parallel with a trend to a decline in age-adjusted stroke, there has also been a trend to a decline in age-adjusted incidence of dementia.[3–5] In the Framingham Heart Study,[5] the 5-year risk of dementia declined by 44 percent between the late 1970s and late 2010s (from 3.6 per hundred to 2 per hundred participants). The most notable differences were a decline in baseline blood pressures (from $137 \pm 19/76 \pm 10$ to $131 \pm 18/70 \pm 10$ mmHg), and an increase in the use of lipid-lowering agents, from none to 43 percent of participants.

Although there are trials under way with disease-modifying agents directed at amyloid and tau proteins, and advances in imaging of amyloid with positron emission tomography show promise for future developments in those avenues of therapy,[6] it is already possible to reduce the risk of dementia by preventing stroke. Delaying dementia reduces the incidence and prevalence of dementia, because at the advanced age at which the risk of dementia is high, patients may die before they become demented. Brookmeyer et al[7] estimated that a two-year delay would reduce prevalence of dementia by 22 percent, and a five-year delay by 47 percent. Alzheimer disease and cerebral infarction interact importantly, and the interaction appears to be bidirectional. In the Nun Study,[8] even one or two small infarctions at the base of the brain increased twenty-fold the likelihood that Alzheimer pathology found at autopsy had been expressed as dementia during life. Conversely, the presence of high levels of amyloid in a rat model with injection of Aβ 25–35 markedly increased the size of infarctions and areas of inflammation, and impaired cognitive function, after infarction induced by injection of endothelin.[9] Mechanisms underlying interaction of amyloid, inflammation, stroke, and dementia were reviewed in 2014.[10]

Furthermore, a very high proportion of patients with any form of dementia have cerebrovascular disease.[11,12] Stroke is eminently preventable; approximately 80 percent of recurrent stroke can be prevented by a combination of diet, smoking cessation, blood pressure control, lipid lowering, antiplatelet agents or anticoagulants as indicated, and appropriate carotid endarterectomy. De Bruijn et al[14] reported from the Rotterdam study, a prospective population-based study, that in the extended cohort approximately a third of dementia would have been avoidable by lifestyle changes and elimination of cardiovascular risk factors. This chapter will focus on preventing dementia by preventing stroke.

Lifestyle Change

Physicians tend to underestimate the importance of lifestyle change. In the U.S. Health Professionals Study, women who followed all five healthy lifestyle choices had an 80 percent reduction of stroke in primary prevention.[15] Perhaps because Swedish people follow a healthier lifestyle, healthy lifestyle choices reduced risk of stroke by "only" 60 percent in Swedish women;[16] however, in high-risk primary prevention, a healthy lifestyle reduced risk of cardiovascular events in Swedish men by 80 percent.[17]

Apart from diet, which will be discussed below, a number of lifestyle changes have the potential to delay cognitive decline: exercise, moderate alcohol intake, and smoking cessation are all important. The Finnish Geriatric Intervention Study to Prevent Cognitive Impairment and Disability (FINGER)[18] recruited 1260 individuals aged 60–77 with a Dementia Risk Score of at least 6 points and cognition at the mean level or slightly lower than expected for age. The participants were randomized to usual community care versus a program of exercise, diet, and monitoring of cardiovascular risk factors. All participants received advice at baseline about healthy diet and exercise, and both groups had the same number of study visits with the nurse and the physician. The intervention group received, in addition, three individual sessions with the nutritionist, and seven to nine group sessions emphasizing exercise and approaches to improving lifestyle. The nutritional advice was this:

> Participants were advised to consume a diet with 10–20 percent of daily energy from proteins, 25–35 percent daily energy from fat (<10 percent from saturated plus trans fatty acids, 10–20 percent from monounsaturated fatty acids, and 5–10 percent from polyunsaturated fatty acids [including 2·5–3 g/day of omega-3 fatty acids]), 45–55 percent daily energy from carbohydrates (<10 percent from refined sugar), 25–35 g/day of dietary fibre, less than 5 g/day of salt, and less than 5 percent daily energy from alcohol. Energy intake facilitating 5–10 percent reduction in body weight was recommended only if necessary after taking into account BMI, health status, age, and diet of the participant. These goals were achieved by recommendation of high consumption of fruit and vegetables, consumption of whole grain cereal products and low-fat milk and meat products, limiting of sucrose intake to less than 50 g/day, use of vegetable margarine and rapeseed oil instead of butter, and fish consumption at least two portions per week.

Two-year assessments were available in 88 percent of participants; those assigned to the intervention arm had significantly better outcomes with regard to the total cognitive score, executive function, and processing speed, with slightly better memory scores that did not reach significance.

Nutrition

Mediterranean Diet

The diet for which there is the strongest evidence for vascular prevention is the Mediterranean diet from the island of Crete. Although it is possible that a vegan diet could be as or more beneficial than a Cretan Mediterranean diet, there are no large well-conducted randomized trials testing that hypothesis. A key reason is probably that, particularly in Western countries, it would be very difficult to achieve compliance. The Mediterranean diet, which is more palatable, is high in beneficial oils such as olive oil and Canola oil, with 40 percent of calories from fat;[19] it is high in fruits, vegetables, lentils, beans, and nuts, and much lower in cholesterol and animal fat than a Western diet. In a retrospective, Ancel Keys, the head of the Seven Countries Study that initially showed the benefit of this diet, described it as follows: "The heart of this diet is mainly vegetarian, and differs from American and northern European diets in that it is much lower in meat and dairy products and uses fruit for dessert."[20]

There is no doubt that a Mediterranean diet significantly reduces the risk of stroke. In the Lyon Diet Heart Study, a secondary prevention trial in survivors of myocardial infarction, the Mediterranean diet reduced cardiovascular events by more than 60 percent in 4 years, compared with a "prudent Western diet" that corresponded to a low fat diet.[21] That effect was twice the effect of simvastatin in the contemporaneous Scandinavian Simvastatin Survival Study (a 40 percent reduction of events in six years). More recently, the Spanish Mediterranean diet study[22] found in high-risk primary prevention that a Mediterranean diet supplemented by mixed nuts reduced stroke by 47 percent, compared to a low fat diet. The authors also reported that the Mediterranean diet reduced cognitive decline.[23] Safouris et al reviewed the reduction of cognitive decline by the Mediterranean diet in 2015.[24]

Dietary issues that deserve special mention are the consumption of cholesterol and egg yolk. Recent recommendations that limits to intake of dietary cholesterol be dropped are probably largely the result of the inordinate success of the sustained and well-funded campaign of propaganda mounted by the egg industry after a conviction for false advertising.[25] As reviewed in Spence, Jenkins, and Davignon,[26] it has been known for many years that dietary cholesterol caused atherosclerosis in animal models, and increased cardiovascular risk in human epidemiological studies; there are good reasons for the long-standing recommendation that cholesterol intake should be less than 200 mg per day.[27] One large egg yolk contains more than 200 mg of cholesterol, so egg yolks are clearly not to be recommended. The egg propaganda rests on a red herring, and a half-truth. The red herring is the misplaced focus on fasting lipids. Diet is not about the fasting state; it is about the post-prandial state.[28] For ~ 4 hours after a high-fat/high cholesterol meal there is oxidative stress, endothelial dysfunction, and arterial inflammation.[26] Egg consumption increases carotid plaque burden by ~ 60 percent as much as smoking,[29] and the effect is additive.[30] Besides the high cholesterol content of egg yolk, the phosphatidylcholine in egg yolk (~ 250 mg in a large egg) is converted by the intestinal microbiome to trimethylamine, which in turn is oxidized to trimethylamine oxide (TMAO).[31] In animal models, TMAO causes atherosclerosis.[31] In patients referred for coronary angiography, TMAO levels after a test dose of two hard-boiled eggs strongly predicted cardiovascular risk: patients in the top quartile of TMAO had a 2.5-fold increase in the 3-year risk of stroke, myocardial infarction, or death.[32] The diet to be recommended for prevention of stroke and dementia would therefore be a Cretan Mediterranean diet, with limitation of the intake of cholesterol, and would prefer egg whites[27] or egg white-based substitutes to whole eggs. As egg whites are a good source of protein, patients can be encouraged to make omelets, frittatas, and even egg salad sandwiches from egg white-based substitutes.[33]

Vitamin B12

A key issue in nutrition for prevention of dementia is metabolic B12 deficiency. With folate fortification in North America, folate deficiency has been virtually eliminated. However, metabolic B12 deficiency is far commoner than most physicians suppose. The problem is that a serum B12 level in the "normal" range (commonly ~ 160–600 pmol/L) is commonly thought by most physicians to exclude B12 deficiency. However, only ~ 6–20 percent of the total serum B12 is active. In order to determine metabolic adequacy of B12, it is necessary to measure holotranscobalamin, or to measure one of the metabolites that is elevated in the presence of inadequate active B12: methylmalonic acid (MMA), which is specific for B12 deficiency, or in folate-replete subjects, total homocysteine (tHcy).[34] In both the NHANES study and the Hordaland study, the serum B12 level below which levels of tHcy and MMA begin to rise is 400 pmol/L. Thus, within the "normal" range of total serum B12, metabolic B12 deficiency is common. Approximately 20 percent of the elderly have B12 deficiency,[35] and among patients attending a stroke prevention clinic, 30 percent of patients above age 70 had metabolic B12 deficiency.[36]

Metabolic B12 deficiency probably accounts for the finding that vitamin B12 was more effective in reducing brain atrophy and reducing the decline of cognitive function among participants with elevated tHcy, in the VITACOG study (Figure 8.3).

Metabolic B12 deficiency is important for several reasons: it contributes to neuropathy, myelopathy, and dementia, and elevates levels of tHcy. High levels of tHcy are an important risk factor for stroke; particularly cardioembolic stroke. There is a "perfect storm" in the conjunction of the aging of the population, the increase in the risk of atrial fibrillation with age, the increase in tHcy with age, and the decline of renal function with age. In the Framingham study, the proportion of strokes attributable to atrial fibrillation increased from 1.5 percent at age 50 to 23.5 percent at age 80–89. In my stroke prevention clinic, the proportion of patients with tHcy above 14 μmol/L (a level associated with increased coagulation) rises from 10 percent at age 35 to 40 percent at age 80. Some of this is due to metabolic B12 deficiency, but a substantial proportion of the rise in tHcy with age is due to a decline in renal function. Figure 8.1 shows the decline in estimated

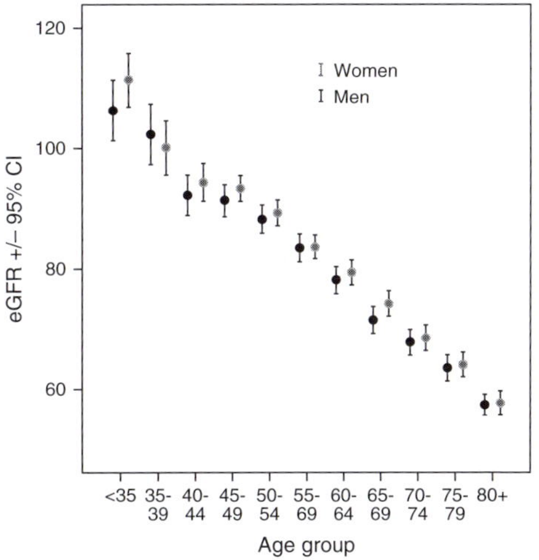

Figure 8.1 Decline in renal function with age Glomerular filtration rate (estimated by the CKD-EPI equation) declines markedly with age in both sexes, among patients attending a stroke prevention clinic. (Reproduced by permission from: Spence JD, Urquhart BL, Bang H. Effect of renal impairment on atherosclerosis: only partially mediated by homocysteine. Nephrol Dial Transplant. 2015.)

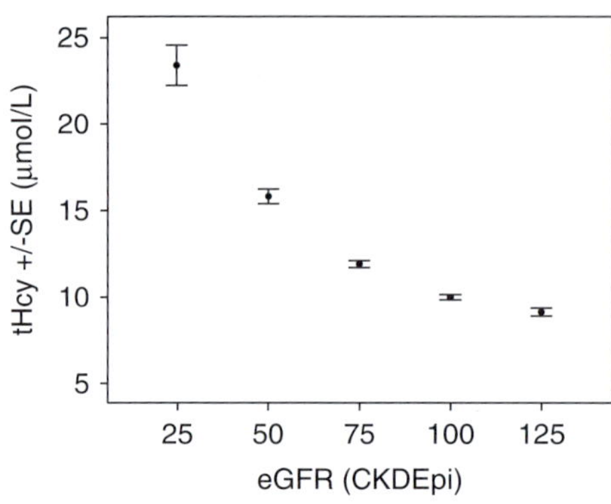

Figure 8.2 Levels of plasma total homocysteine (tHcy) are markedly increased with renal impairment. Glomerular filtration rate was estimated by the CKD-EPI equations. Data are from patients referred to the Stroke Prevention & Atherosclerosis Research Centre, Robarts Research Institute, Western University, London, Canada. n = 1758.

glomerular filtration rate (eGFR) with age, and Figure 8.2 shows the rise in tHcy with decline in eGFR.

In 2006, it was widely believed that vitamin therapy to lower homocysteine was "dead", because the Vitamin Intervention for Stroke Prevention (VISP) trial[37] and the NORVIT trial failed to show benefit of B vitamin therapy. The authors of the HOPE-2 trial, being cardiologists and therefore innocent of the cerebral circulation, said essentially that because they could not think of a biological difference between stroke and myocardial infarction, the significant reduction of stroke that they observed[38] should be regarded as a chance finding. However, the issues are more complex than they seemed;[39] clinical trials are a blunt instrument for studying vascular biology.

The null result of the VISP trial could be explained on several grounds: 1) Folate fortification of the grain supply in North America began at the same time the study was initiated, thus negating the benefit of folic acid. 2) We did not use a placebo; in the hope of limiting noncompliance to the assigned therapy, participants were given low-dose or a high-dose vitamin tablets containing folic acid, pyridoxine, and cyanocobalamin. 3) Because participants would be receiving some folic acid in the low-dose arm of the study, and there was concern that this might mask B12 deficiency, participants with serum B12 levels below the normal range were given monthly B12 injections, regardless of their treatment assignment, thus negating the benefit of B12 in the very patients who would have benefited most. 4) The high-dose vitamin contained only 400 mcg of cyanocobalamin, which was subsequently shown to be too low a dose for absorption of B12 by elderly patients with serum B12 in the lowest quartile. (The HOPE-2 trial, which showed a significant, 23 percent, reduction of stroke was the first to use 1000 mcg of B12, which is an adequate dose for elderly persons with impaired B12 absorption.)

The subgroup analysis of VISP,[40] for reasons explained above, excluded participants who received injections of B12; it also excluded, for a reason that turned out in retrospect to be wrong, participants with renal impairment: those with an eGFR in the lowest decile, which turned out to be 48 mL/min/1.73 m². (The reason for excluding patients with low eGFR was that we thought, on the basis of an earlier study in dialysis patients showing no difference between 1mg and 5mg daily of folate, that patients with renal impairment would not respond to B vitamins.) We stratified participants at the median baseline serum B12 level to reflect adequacy of absorption of B12 above vs. below that level (322 pmol/L). As shown in Figure 8.4, there was a 34 percent reduction in stroke, myocardial infarction or

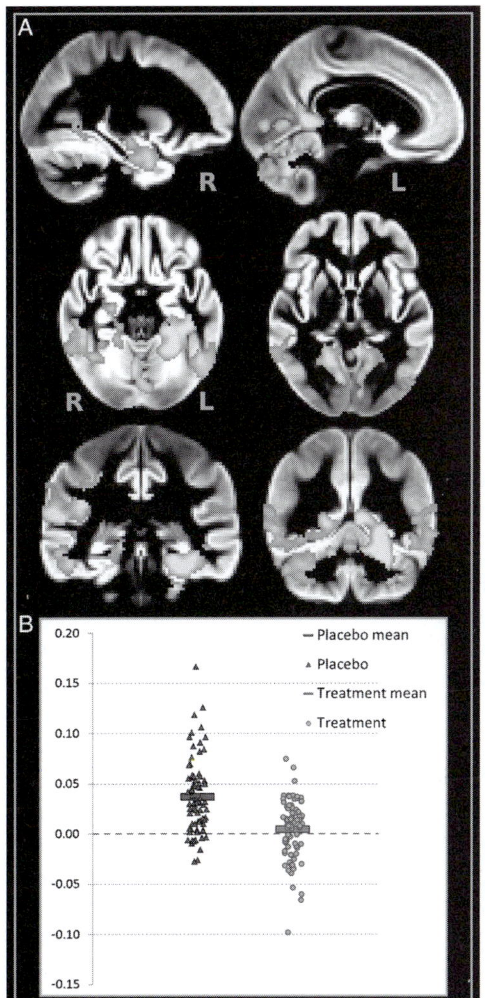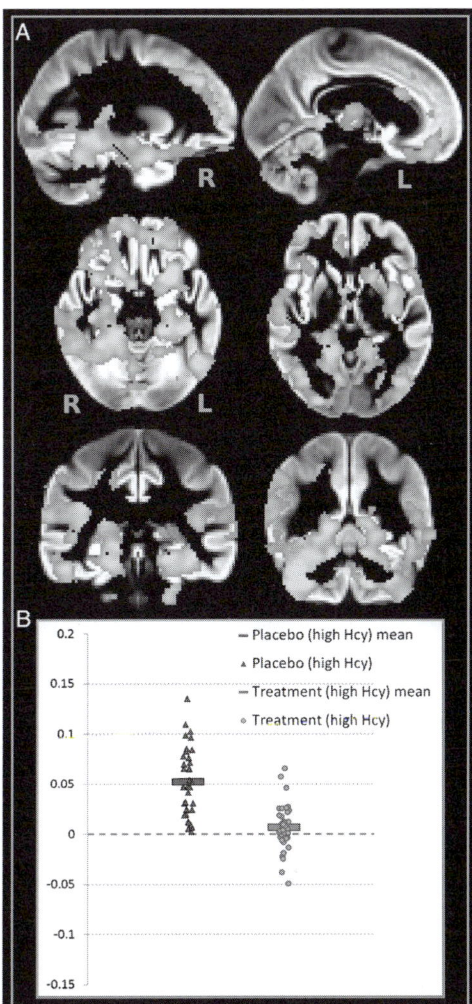

Figure 8.3 B-vitamin therapy reduces loss of gray matter (GM) in Alzheimer disease–related regions of the brain in elderly individuals with mild cognitive impairment.
B-vitamin treatment was more effective in participants with higher tHcy levels ($P < .05$ FEW corrected). (A) Brain regions in green (color is seen in the online version of the chapter) demonstrate where B-vitamin treatment significantly reduces GM loss in participants with high tHcy levels (>11.06 µmol/L) at baseline. (B) Percentage of GM loss for each of the 77 participants with high tHcy level: the placebo group (n = 35) showed an average loss of 5.2% (±3.4) of GM volume over 2 years, whereas the Bvitamin group (n =42) showed an average loss of 0.6% (±2.1). (Reproduced by permission of the National Academy of Sciences of the United States of America, from: Douaud G, Refsum H, de Jager CA, Jacoby R, Nichols TE, Smith SM et al. Preventing Alzheimer's disease–related gray matter atrophy by B-vitamin treatment. Proc Natl Acad Sci U S A. 2013;110:9523–8).

death among participants with a baseline serum B12 above the median given high-dose vitamins, compared with participants with a serum B12 below the median given low-dose B vitamins. The Logrank test was significant for all for all four groups.

Subsequently, we carried out a randomized trial in patients with diabetic nephropathy, comparing placebo to high-dose B vitamins containing 1000 mcg of cyanocobalamin.

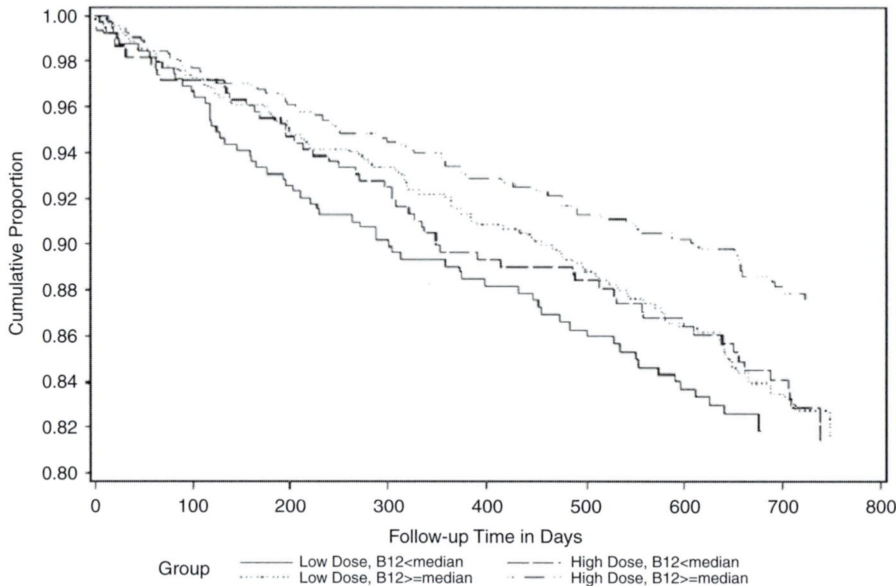

Figure 8.4 Kaplan–Meier survival free of combined stroke, death, and coronary events by baseline B12 stratum. Participants were stratified above or below the median level of 322 pmol/L, and by treatment group (high-dose versus low-dose vitamin therapy); P<0.02 from log-rank test comparing all 4 groups. Those with a serum B12 above the median, who were randomized to high-dose vitamins had a 34 percent reduction of events compared with those with a serum B12 below the median who were randomized to low-dose B vitamins. (Permission granted by Wolters Kluver to reproduce from: Spence JD, Bang H, Chambless LE, Stampfer MJ. Vitamin Intervention For Stroke Prevention trial: an efficacy analysis. *Stroke.* 2005;36:2404–2409.)

To our surprise and dismay, we found that high-dose B vitamins accelerated the decline of renal function, and doubled the proportion of patients with events.[41] All the events occurred among participants with a GFR below 50 mL/min/1.73 m^2,[42] very close to the level used to exclude participants from the VISP efficacy analysis. At the time, it was hypothesized that either cyanocobalamin or folic acid may have been harmful. Now in the light of the Chinese Primary Stroke Prevention Trial, which showed a significant reduction of stroke and improvement of renal function even among participants with low eGFR with folic acid, it is apparent that the harm in VISP was from cyanocobalamin. Reasons why it is probably the cyanide in cyanocobalamin that caused the harm were reviewed in 2015:[34] 1) Cyanide consumes hydrogen sulfide, a nitric oxide antagonist, in the formation of thiocyanate. 2) Patients with renal failure have high levels of thiocyanate, which increases oxidation of LDL cholesterol. 3) Methylcobalamin lowers both tHcy and levels of asymmetric dimethylarginine (ADMA), a nitric oxide antagonist. 4) Cyanocobalamin does not lower levels of ADMA. 5) Cyanocobalamin is not effective in alcohol-tobacco amblyopia (a condition in which cyanide is important), whereas hydroxycobalamin is effective. All of the foregoing indicates that we should be using methylcobalamin rather than cyanocobalamin, particularly in patients with renal impairment (which essentially includes the elderly).

The marked increase in cardiovascular risk with renal failure is not all attributable to elevation of tHcy. A mediation study[43] indicated that tHcy accounts for only 12 percent of the effect of eGFR on carotid plaque burden. Other uremic toxins include ADMA, thiocyanate (from tobacco, cyanocobalamin, and other sources), and metabolic products of the intestinal microbiome, including trimethylamine N-oxide (TMAO) (from carnitine, lecithin), indoxyl sulfate (from tryptophan) indole 3-acetic acid (from tryptophan), and p-cresyl sulfate (from tyrosine). Thus patients with renal impairment should restrict their intake of red meat (with 4 times as much carnitine as white flesh), and should be particularly careful to avoid egg yolk. Approaches to reducing these uremic toxins include more intensive dialysis, such as daily overnight dialysis, the use of pure carbon administered orally to absorb uremic toxins in the intestine, and possibly the use of thiols to remove uremic toxins from plasma proteins to make them more dialyzable.[43]

Stroke Prevention: Medical and Surgical Interventions

Blood Pressure Control

Evidence that lowering blood pressure reduces the risk of dementia was reviewed in 2013.[44] Controlling blood pressure is perhaps the most effective medical intervention for stroke prevention, with the potential to reduce stroke by 40–50 percent. Most strokes (~ 90 percent) occur in patients with uncontrolled hypertension. The strokes that are prevented are those caused directly by high blood pressure, damaging the arterioles at the base of the brain, in the distribution called by Hachinski the "vascular centrencephalon" (Figure 8.5). In that phylogenetically ancient part of the brain, short arteries branch off perpendicularly from large arteries, and because they have few branches, deliver high blood pressure directly to the arterioles. This leads to hyaline degeneration and fibrinoid necrosis, causing lacunar infarctions when the arterioles occlude, and intracerebral hemorrhage when they rupture. Controlling hypertension will only prevent lacunar infarctions and intracerebral hemorrhages in the vascular centrencephalon. Most lobar hemorrhages are due to amyloid angiopathy, and small subcortical ischemic lesions over the convexity, seen on MRI as white matter intensities (WMI) are probably due to low diastolic pressure, particularly in patients with wide pulse pressure due to arterial stiffness. In the setting of high blood pressure, with a pressure of 190/110 in the internal carotid, blood pressure in the vascular centrencephalon is 180/100, whereas in the parietal convexity it drops to 117/68 mmHg.[45] Black suggests that periventricular WMIs are attributable to venous congestion.

Improving Blood Pressure Control

Despite all the evidence that lowering blood pressure prevents stroke, hypertension remains poorly controlled. Figure 8.6 shows that among patients referred to an Urgent TIA Clinic between 2002 and 2012, blood pressure control at the time of referral, reflecting community practice, remained poor: half of patients had systolic pressures above 140, and 20 percent had pressures above 90 mmHg. Reasons for poor blood pressure control include therapeutic inertia, and diagnostic inertia.[46] Therapeutic inertia probably results from a combination of patient reluctance to take medication, the mistaken belief that white coat hypertension is benign, and competition for attention of the physician of comorbidities such as diabetes, arthritis, pain, and other chronic conditions. Therapeutic inertia can be overcome: in the North American Symptomatic Carotid Endarterectomy Trial, investigators received a letter insisting they follow the protocol, whenever a participant's blood pressure medication was not increased at any visit at which the blood pressure exceeded the target level. This reduced intracranial hemorrhage (including subarachnoid and lobar hemorrhages, which are not attributable to hypertension) to 0.4 percent of stroke.

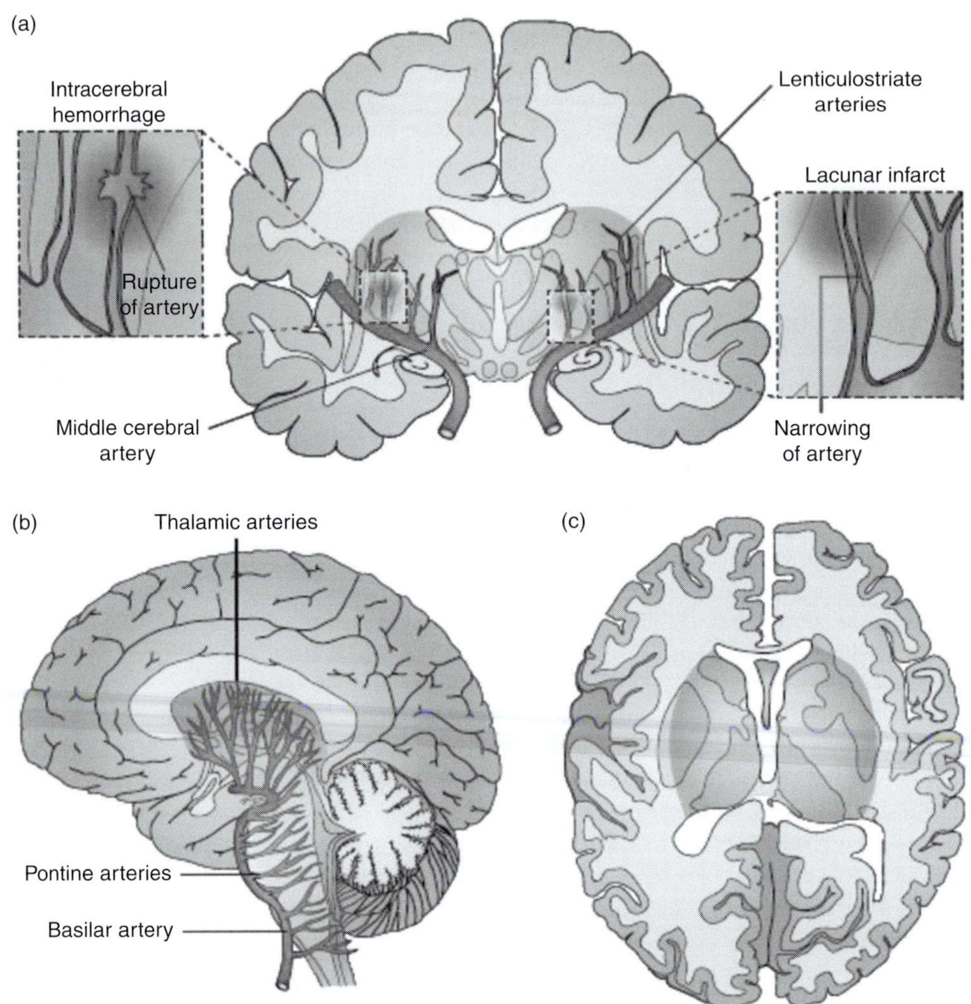

Figure 8.5 Pathophysiology of lacunar and haemorrhagic stroke.
End arteries originate perpendicularly from the major vessels of the anterior and posterior circulation, without substantial collaterals from adjacent arteries. These arteries are particularly vulnerable to arterial hypertension, which causes fibrinoid degeneration and microaneurysms of the vessel wall, and result in narrowing (lacunar ischemic infarct) or rupture (intracerebral hemorrhage) of arteries. End arteries supply the vascular centrencephalon (blue region), which includes phylogenetically older parts of the brain (including the brainstem, basal ganglia, and thalamus), and adjacent white matter: a) Coronal view. b) Sagittal view. c) Axial view. (Reproduced by permission of Nature from: Sörös P, Whitehead S, Spence JD, Hachinski V. Antihypertensive treatment can prevent stroke and cognitive decline. Nat Rev Neurol. 2013 Mar;9(3):174–8.)

Diagnostic inertia (failure of physicians to investigate the underlying cause of resistant hypertension) seems to be particularly intransigent. Despite the fine print in hypertension guidelines, recommending measurement of investigations including plasma renin and aldosterone in patients with resistant hypertension, physicians for the most part persist in prescribing the same cookie-cutter therapy to all their patients, as if they were all the same. This is particularly a problem in black patients. African-Americans have twice the risk of stroke, and the strokes they

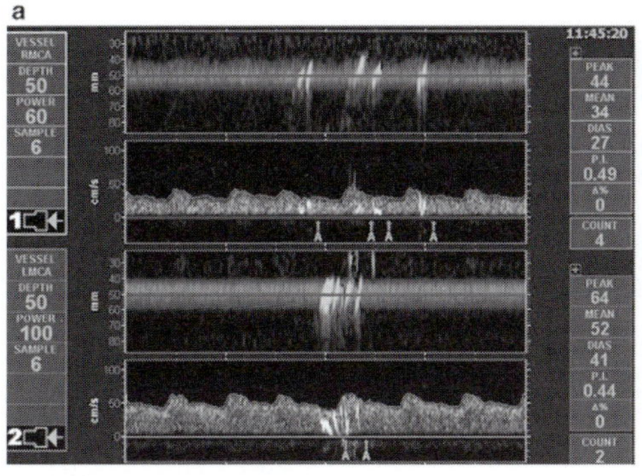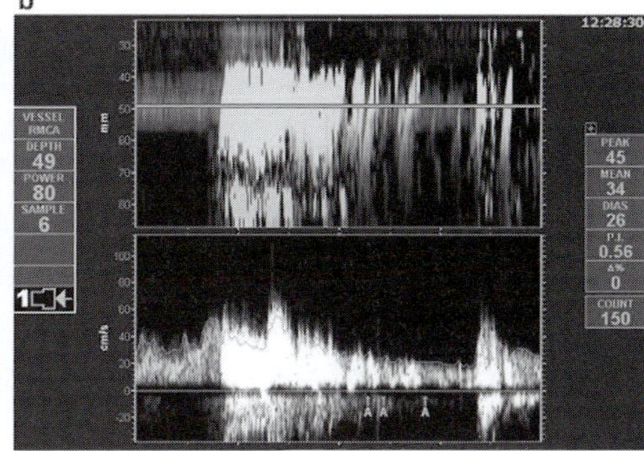

Figure 8.6 Microemboli during carotid stenting.
Showers of emboli of atheromatous debris occur commonly (even usually) during carotid stenting, and can be observed by transcranial Doppler. The upper row on each side is the M-mode image from the middle cerebral artery; the lower shows high-intensity transit signals in the Doppler channel. Panel A shows microemboli in both middle cerebral arteries (4 on the right and 2 on the left), while the aortic arch was being crossed; Panel B shows 150 microemboli in the right middle cerebral artery during stenting of the right internal carotid artery, during one cardiac cycle and the beginning of the next. (Courtesy of Dr. Claudio Muñoz; permission was granted by Springer to reproduce from: Spence JD. Management of patients with an asymptomatic carotid stenosis – medical management, endovascular treatment, or carotid endarterectomy? *Current Neurology & Neuroscience.* 2016;(1):3).

have are more likely to be hypertensive strokes (lacunar infarctions and hypertensive intracerebral hemorrhages). This is true even though African-Americans are more likely to have their hypertension diagnosed, more likely to have it treated, and more likely to have it treated more intensively.[47]

Reasons for this were reviewed in 2012:[48] black patients are known to have lower levels of plasma renin, due to genetic causes of salt and water retention, that may have conferred a selective advantage in hot arid conditions. Primary aldosteronism accounts for ~ 20 percent of resistant hypertension and is more common in African-Americans. Variants of Liddle syndrome (mutations of a renal tubular sodium channel that cause salt and water retention and excretion of potassium) were present in 20 percent of the Khoi San people of the Kalahari, 9 percent of Zulu, and 6 percent of all patients attending a hypertension clinic in Cape Town, South Africa. A different variant was found in 5 percent of black patients in London, UK, and a Liddle phenotype (low renin and aldosterone) was found in 6 percent of patients attending a Veteran's Administration clinic in Louisiana.

Recent U.S. hypertension guidelines recommending higher pressures than in the past, and Canadian guidelines recommending that white coat hypertension not be treated, have been overturned by the publication of the Systolic Pressure Intervention Trial (SPRINT),[49] which showed that lower pressures are better. However, a note of caution is warranted. The J curve is probably explained by cuff artefact in blood pressure measurement that results in very low diastolic pressures when patients whose cuff pressure is much higher than the true intra-arterial pressure are treated on the basis of the falsely elevated cuff pressure.[46] There is a marked drop in blood pressure from the base of the brain to small arterioles over the convexity.[45] In the Atherosclerosis Risk in Communities (ARIC) study, participants with a wide pulse pressure and a diastolic pressure below 60 mmHg had an increased risk of coronary artery disease.[50] Stiff arteries are predictive of cognitive decline,[51] and a wide pulse pressure (which is due to arterial stiffness) is predictive of small white matter intensities over the convexity.[52] It is possible that

Table 8.1 Physiologically individualized therapy* based on renin/aldosterone profile

	Primary hyper-aldosteronism	Liddle's syndrome and variants (renal Na+ channel mutations)	Renal/renovascular
Renin	Low**	Low	High
Aldosterone	High**	Low	High
Primary treatment	Aldosterone antagonist (spironolactone or eplerenone) Amiloride for men where eplerenone is not available (rarely surgery)	Amiloride	Angiotensin receptor blocker or renin inhibitor*** (rarely revascularization)

   * It should be stressed that this approach is suitable for tailoring medical therapy in resistant hypertensives; further investigation would be required to justify adrenalectomy or renal revascularization

  ** Levels of plasma renin and aldosterone must be interpreted in the light of the medication the patient is taking at the time of sampling. In a patient taking an angiotensin receptor blocker (which would elevate renin and lower aldosterone), a plasma renin that is in the low normal range for that laboratory, with a plasma aldosterone in the high normal range, probably represents primary hyperaldosteronism, for the purposes of adjusting medical therapy.

*** Angiotensin converting enzyme inhibitors are less effective because of aldosterone escape via non-ACE pathways such as chymase and cathepsin.

(Permission was granted by Elsevier to reproduce from: Spence JD. Lessons from Africa: the importance of measuring plasma renin and aldosterone in resistant hypertension. *Can J Cardiol.* 2012;28(3):254–7.)

elderly patients with stiff arteries may be at increased risk of cognitive decline from diastolic hypotension if their true diastolic pressure is much lower than that measured by a cuff. It may be prudent to avoid diastolic pressures below 60 mmHg. In this regard, beta blockers may be a problem, because bradycardia, by increasing stroke volume, widens pulse pressure.

Inadequate blood pressure control is an important remediable cause of strokes and dementia, and the fault lies at the feet of physicians whose patients suffer from diagnostic inertia.

Table 8.1 presents an algorithm for detecting the underlying cause of resistant hypertension, and identifying the most appropriate therapy. Patients with primary aldosteronism (which is commonly due to bilateral adrenocortical hyperplasia) seldom need adrenalectomy; they should be treated with aldosterone antagonists (spironolactone or eplerenone). Amiloride is the specific treatment for Liddle variants, and patients with renal hypertension should be treated with angiotensin receptor antagonists or renin inhibitors. Severe renovascular hypertension may require revascularization. This algorithm was tested in a trial in Africa; physiological treatment based on phenotyping by renin and aldosterone levels markedly improved blood pressure control, compared to usual care.[53]

Treatment of Diabetes

There is some evidence that control of diabetes may slow cognitive decline.[18,54] It is likely that this may be related to reduction of stroke, particularly stroke from intracranial stenosis, which is commoner in diabetes. Key issues are weight loss, exercise, and maintenance of a normal or near-normal glycosylated hemoglobin. Pioglitazone, a Peroxisome proliferator-activated receptor agonist that reduces insulin resistance, reduces the risk of stroke, and new antidiabetic therapies offer promise of future improvements.

Antiplatelet Therapy and Anticoagulation

There have been recent important advances in both antiplatelet therapy and anticoagulation. In 2013, it was reported[55] that enteric coating of aspirin resulted in pseudoresistance to the antiplatelet effects of aspirin; this may account for the longstanding controversy about "aspirin resistance." Dual antiplatelet therapy with aspirin and clopidogrel, long known to be more efficacious in acute coronary syndrome, now has better evidence in stroke. A large Chinese study showed better outcomes with dual antiplatelet therapy, and the SAMPPRIS trial in intracranial stenosis used this combination. Evidence from studies of microemboli with transcranial Doppler show reduce microemboli with dual antiplatelet therapy in both intracranial stenosis and carotid stenosis.

An important problem with clopidogrel is that it is a prodrug requiring activation by CYP2C19, and there are important interactions that prevent its activation, notably with proton pump inhibitors. An exception appears to be pantoprazole. Fortunately, these problems will be obviated by new antiplatelet agents that appear to be more efficacious, and ticagrelor in particular is not subject to the interactions affecting clopidogrel and prasugrel.

The arrival of new oral anticoagulants (NOACs), which include apixaban, dabigatran, edoxaban, and rivaroxaban (in alphabetical order), has revolutionized the management of patients with known or suspected cardioembolic stroke. This comes at an opportune time, as with better treatment of hypertension and lowering of LDL cholesterol, the proportion of strokes due to emboli from the heart has doubled between 2002 and 2012; in a Canadian Urgent TIA clinic population, this increased from approximately a quarter to half of strokes. It is absolutely clear that anticoagulation is necessary for atrial fibrillation; antiplatelet agents do not prevent polymerization of fibrin that is the basis for the formation of "red thrombus" – clots that form in the setting of stasis, such as in a deep vein, atrial appendage, or areas of ventricular dyskinesia. Fear of anticoagulation with warfarin on the part of both patients ("I don't want to take rat poison, and I don't want to have frequent blood tests") and physicians (who overemphasize in their memory the most recent catastrophic hemorrhage in a patient taking warfarin) was misplaced: a French study calculated that some 200 falls on warfarin would be needed to equal the risk of not taking warfarin in atrial fibrillation. In the AVERROES study, there was no higher risk of severe bleeding on apixaban than on aspirin, so the assumption on which past reluctance to anticoagulate patients, and to prefer antiplatelet agents, is now invalid. This means that everything has changed, and we should probably be anticoagulating not only patients with established cardioembolic sources such as atrial fibrillation, but also patients in whom cardioembolic stroke is strongly suspected.

Clinical clues to cardioembolic stroke include negative features such as the absence of hypertension, atherosclerosis, and other causes of stroke ("cryptogenic stroke"), and positive clues to a cardioembolic source such as multiple territory cortical events. A patient who has a left homonymous hemianopsia one day, and then an episode of aphasia and right arm clumsiness on another day has probably had cardioembolic events. The hypothesis that patients with embolic stroke of unknown significance ("ESUS") should be anticoagulated is being tested in a clinical trial.

Table 8.2 Clinical pharmacology of new oral anticoagulants

	Apixaban	Dabigatran	Edoxaban	Rivaroxaban
Inhibitor of	Factor Xa	Factor IIa	Factor Xa	Factor Xa
Regimen	Twice daily	Twice daily	Once daily	Once daily with food
Bioavailability (%)	~ 50%	~6%	~60%	~ 80%
Terminal half-life	8–15 hours	12–14 hours	10–14 hours	5–13 hours
Renal elimination (%)	~ 25%	~ 85%	~ 50%	~ 33%
Drug interactions*	CYP3A4 and P-gp	P-gp	P-gp	CYP3A4 and P-gp

P-gp = P-glycoprotein; drug efflux transport protein
Moderate/strong inhibitors: grapefruit; antiarrhthymics: quinidine, verapamil, amiodarone.
Antifungals: ketoconazole, itraconazole; Immunosuppressants: tacrolimus, cyclosporine.
Protease inhibitor antivirals: ritonavir, indinavir, nelfinavir, saquinavir.
CYP3A4 = cytochrome P450 3A4; drug oxidation in the intestine and liver
Strong inhibitors: Grapefruit (juice or fruit; even one glass; duration more than 24 hours). Protease inhibitor
antivirals: ritonavir, indinavir, nelfinavir, saquinavir. Antibiotics: erythromycin, clarithromycin, telithromycin,
chloramphenicol. Antifungals: ketoconazole, itraconazole. Others: nefazodone, cobicistat, cyclosporine
* It is impossible to remember all drug interactions; when planning to initiate a new drug it is important to look
  up interactions with all other drugs the patient is taking; in a patient already taking a NOAC for whom a new
  drug is intended to be prescribed, it is important to look up the interactions.

Although the manufacturers state that blood testing is not required with the NOACs, this appears not to be the case for dabigatran. There may also be a problem with the once-daily dosing of edoxaban and rivaroxaban, the half-life of which is not materially longer than that of the other agents. A particular problem with dabigatran is that it has a very low bioavailability (6 percent), which means that it is subject to major effects of malabsorption or drug interactions. An example of this principle is simvastatin, which is only 5 percent bioavailable because during absorption 95 percent of the drug is metabolized in the intestinal wall by CYP3A4. This means that total inhibition of CYP3A4 could theoretically increase blood levels twenty-fold, and indeed grapefruit juice, a strong inhibitor of intestinal CYP3A4 increases simvastatin blood levels (AUC) fifteen-fold, with the potential to cause rhabdomyolysis. Table 8.2 shows some of the clinical pharmacology of the NOACs.

Treatment of Atherosclerosis

Intensive treatment with lipid-lowering drugs can not only halt the progression of atherosclerosis; it can cause regression of atherosclerosis and stabilize plaques. This is particularly important for patients with large artery strokes. The benefit of high-dose atorvastatin in secondary prevention was underestimated in the SPARCL trial because of inclusion of many patients with strokes that were lacunar, and by a high rate of crossover from placebo to statin therapy (approximately 25 percent of patients), with an intention-to-treat analysis. Although atorvastatin only reduced stroke by ~ 16 percent in the overall study population, it reduced stroke by ~ 30 percent in patients with large artery disease, and because of the crossover rate this would have been higher.

High-dose statins may cause myopathy and slightly increase the risk of diabetes; the mechanism is probably reduction of muscle levels of CoQ10, by the same action that lowers cholesterol. A useful strategy for patients with statin myopathy, diabetes, or prediabetes is to use a moderate dose of statin in combination with ezetimibe, a specific inhibitor of intestinal receptors for absorption of cholesterol. Ezetimibe and statins are synergistic; 10 mg of ezetimibe with 10mg of atorvastatin has the same LDL-lowering effect as 80 mg daily of atorvastatin, but with less adverse effects. A recent important development in lipid lowering is the approval of treatments to block the action of PCSK9, an enzyme that breaks down LDL receptors. Injections of antibodies to PCSK9 result in prolonged persistence of LDL receptors, and lower LDL cholesterol by ~50 percent over and above the effect of statins. Unfortunately, these biological agents are very expensive; it is to be hoped that an affordable small molecule antagonist to PCSK9 might become available before long.

The potential of intensive LDL-lowering was observed among patients with asymptomatic stenosis, comparing patients referred to a stroke prevention clinic before and after 2003, when a more intensive regimen called "treating arteries instead of treating risk factors"[56] was implemented. The rate of plaque progression was significantly reduced, microemboli on transcranial Doppler were reduced by three-fourths (suggesting stabilization of plaque), and, more importantly, events were markedly reduced: the 2-year risk of stroke or myocardial infarction declined by more than 80 percent.[57] It is probably not coincidental that ezetimibe was released on the market in 2003; a study of patients with serial measurement of carotid plaque burden for two years before and two years after initiation of ezetimibe showed plaque regression after initiation of ezetimibe.[58]

Appropriate Carotid Endarterectomy and Stenting

The issues discussed were recently reviewed.[59,60] There is no doubt that most patients with severe symptomatic carotid stenosis will benefit from carotid endarterectomy, when carried out by surgeons with a high volume of cases and low risk (<3 percent): the number needed to treat (NNT) was only 6 for younger patients, and only 3 for patients age 75 and older. Carotid stenting carries approximately twice the risk of stroke or death compared with endarterectomy, so should be reserved for patients with special features such as high medical risk, prior neck surgery with scarring, a high bifurcation, and post-radiation arteriopathy.

Asymptomatic carotid stenosis is a different matter. Even based on the old data from studies carried out ~ 20 years ago, the NNT for asymptomatic stenosis was 83. With modern intensive medical therapy, the risk of ipsilateral stroke has declined to ~ 0.5 percent, so even the promising results of the CREST trial (a 30-day risk of stroke or death of 2.5 percent for stenting and 1.4 percent for endarterectomy, with a 4-year risk of 4.5 percent with stenting and 2.7 percent with endarterectomy) do not justify routine intervention for asymptomatic stenosis. Stenting is more hazardous in older patients with stiff, tortuous arteries. Figure 8.6 shows microemboli detected in the middle cerebral arteries of patients undergoing stenting. A higher proportion of patients have small silent infarctions shown on diffusion-weighted MRI after stenting than after endarterectomy.

It is not legitimate to compare the results in the medical arm of studies carried out 20 years ago with the surgical results of modern studies that had no medical arm. Deplorably, in the United States ~ 90 percent of carotid intervention is for asymptomatic stenosis; this contrasts with ~ 60 percent in Germany and Italy, ~ 15 percent in Canada and Australia (about right), and 0 percent in Denmark. These discrepancies highlight the inappropriateness of practice in the United States and Europe, which can be considered unethical, or worse. A problem that is particular to the United States is that 30 percent of interventionalists performing carotid stenting are cardiologists, and they are performing ~ 50 percent of the procedures. One reason for this may be the failure of cardiologists to understand the protection afforded by the Circle of Willis; they may think that occlusion of a carotid artery would be similar to occlusion of a left main coronary (a ticking time bomb). However, the Circle of Willis is remarkably protective: among 316 patients with a de novo occlusion of an internal carotid artery observed during annual carotid ultrasound examinations, only one (0.3 percent) had a stroke at the time of the occlusion. Thus prevention of occlusion is not a valid indication for endarterectomy.

Fortunately, the few patients with asymptomatic carotid stenosis who could benefit from revascularization can be identified. The best validated method is transcranial Doppler embolus detection. Spence et al reported in 2005 that the 10 percent of patients with asymptomatic stenosis and microemboli on TCD had a 1-year risk of stroke of 15.6 percent, well above the risk of revascularization; however, the 90 percent of patients with no microemboli had only a 1 percent 1-year risk of stroke, so would be more likely to be harmed than helped by endarterectomy (and more so by stenting). That finding was substantiated in a follow-up paper in 468 patients in 2010, and in 467 patients in the international multicenter Asymptomatic Carotid Emboli Study (ACES). Other approaches to identifying high-risk asymptomatic stenosis include identification of ulceration by 3D ultrasound, assessment of cerebral blood flow reserve, intraplaque hemorrhage on MRI and plaque inflammation on positron emission tomography.

Postmenopausal Hormone Replacement Therapy

Whether postmenopausal hormone replacement therapy (HRT) for women might slow cognitive decline is controversial. Although the rationale for the Kronos Early Estrogen Prevention Study (KEEPS)[61] may be sound, the study was probably underpowered; there were only 571 participants, mean age 52 years at inception, and the participants were followed for only four years, so may not have been old enough to detect a possible effect over a longer term. Similarly, the Women's Health Initiative study randomized 1326 women age 50 to 55 to HRT versus placebo, and followed them for seven years, with no significant delay of cognitive decline. The most recent Cochrane review[62] did not support HRT for slowing of cognitive decline.

With regard to male testosterone deficiency, a meta-analysis in 2015[63] reported a significant increase in Alzheimer's disease with testosterone deficiency.

The other side of the coin is the controversial issue of HRT for women and testosterone replacement therapy (TRT) for men, with regard to cardiovascular risk. As reviewed by Spence and Pilote,[64] the issues are more complex than commonly understood (references are omitted from this quotation, as they are available in the source publication):

> There is an abundance of evidence that in animal models estrogen is protective against atherosclerosis. Similarly, there is ample evidence that testosterone deficiency increases the risk of atherosclerotic events. Thus estrogen replacement for women, and testosterone replacement for men, ought to be beneficial. Yet both are widely regarded as being harmful. The issues are more complex than may be generally appreciated.
>
> Although the Women's Health Initiative trial is commonly thought to have put an end to postmenopausal hormone replacement therapy (HRT), a key issue for interpretation of this issue is the question of predisposition to estrogen-induced thrombosis by Factor V Leiden or

other thrombogenic disorders. It is possible that excluding women with Factor V Leiden may avoid many of the thrombotic complications related to estrogen.

Perhaps the best data on thrombogenic effects of estrogen come from a prospective study of oral contraceptive therapy in Denmark that showed a statistically significant increase in the risk of stroke with preparations containing 30–40 mcg of ethinyl estradiol, with relative risks that seem rather high, ranging from 1.3 to 2.2 depending on the progesterone component of the preparation. However, the absolute risk was very small (0.02 percent). This is lower than the risk of stroke during pregnancy and the postpartum period (0.034 percent), so the risks of oral contraception may have been exaggerated. A California study found that 1,015 (0.06 percent) had a thrombotic event (248 strokes, 47 myocardial infarctions and 720 cases of venous thromboembolism). The risk was higher in the first six weeks postpartum than a year later.

Two large trials in women with vascular disease, the Heart and Estrogen/Progestin Replacement study (HERS) and the Women's Estrogen for Stroke Trial (WEST) showed no benefit or harm from HRT with regard to stroke.

The Women's Health Initiative study, a randomized trial of conjugated estrogen 0.625 mg daily vs. placebo in postmenopausal women with hysterectomy, found hazard ratios (95 percent confidence intervals) of 0.91 (0.75–1.12) for coronary disease, 1.39 (1.1–1.77) for stroke, 1.34 (0.87–2.06) for pulmonary embolism, and a reduction of hip fracture: 0.61(0.4 –0.91). However, the excess risk was a "non-significant two events per 10,000 person-years." Thus the hysteria over HRT (pun intended) seems unwarranted. Indeed, the Danish Osteoporosis Prevention Study (DOPS), in recently menopausal healthy women ages 45–58 at inception, found that after 10 years women receiving HRT had a significantly reduced risk of heart failure, myocardial infarction, or death, with no apparent increase in the risk of cancer, venous thromboembolism, or stroke.

There is a similar controversy about testosterone replacement in men. Health Canada recently released an advisory regarding testosterone therapy at www.hc-sc.gc.ca/dhp-mps /medeff/reviews-examens/testosterone-eng.php. It seems to be based largely on a study by Vigen et al. The totality of the literature; suggests that testosterone would probably improve quality of life and reduce cardiovascular risk. Page pointed out that the primary data in the Vigen study actually showed a 50 percent reduction of cardiovascular risk with testosterone replacement before adjustment for some 50 variables.

A key issue for TRT may be adequacy of dosing. A study of 83,010 male veterans with documented low testosterone levels compared men whose testosterone level was normalized with TRT, with men not receiving TRT, and with men receiving inadequate doses of TRT. Utilizing propensity score-weighted Cox proportional hazard models, the authors reported that normalization of testosterone levels was associated with a significant reduction of stroke, myocardial infarction and all-cause mortality.[65]

Thus, it appears likely that HRT for women and TRT for men, by reducing cardiovascular risk, might also reduce the risk of dementia in the long term. Large long-term studies in participants old enough to be at increased risk of dementia would be needed to test this hypothesis.

Summary and Conclusions

The future of preventing dementia holds promise for disease-modifying drugs directed at amyloid and tau proteins. However, because stroke interacts importantly with dementia of all types, it is already possible to reduce the rate of cognitive decline and delay dementia by a number of interventions known to prevent stroke. Lifestyle interventions are far more effective than most physicians assume. It is important to help patients quit smoking, adopt a Mediterranean diet, moderate their alcohol intake, and exercise regularly. Key medical and surgical interventions that reduce the risk of stroke include antiplatelet therapy, anticoagulation, and revascularization in appropriate cases. An important missed opportunity for prevention of stroke is missed metabolic B12 deficiency; treatment with methylcobalamin should be given to patients with a serum total B12 in the low end of the normal range if there is a low level of holotranscobalamin or a high level of methylmalonic acid (or of tHcy in folate-replete patients). Perhaps the biggest potential for preventing dementia is from blood pressure reduction. Individualized therapy based on the physiology of the underlying cause is key to achieving control of resistant hypertension. Time is brain; these measures should all be implemented vigorously and early in patients at risk of dementia.

References

1. Kosteniuk JG, Morgan DG, O'Connell ME, et al. Incidence and prevalence of dementia in linked administrative health data in Saskatchewan, Canada: a retrospective cohort study. *BMC Geriatr.* 2015;**15**:73.

2. The road map to integrated dementia prevention and care. *Lancet Neurol.* 2013;**12** (9):839.

3. Wu YT, Fratiglioni L, Matthews FE, et al. Dementia in western Europe: epidemiological evidence and implications for policy making. *Lancet Neurol.* 2015 ;**15** (1):116–124.

4. Sposato LA, Kapral MK, Fang J, Gill SS, Hackam DG, Cipriano LE, et al. Declining incidence of stroke and dementia: coincidence or prevention opportunity? *JAMA Neurol.* 2015;**72**(12):1529–31.

5. Satizabal CL, Beiser AS, Chouraki V, Chêne G, Dufouil C, Seshadri S. Incidence of dementia over three decades in the Framingham Heart Study. *N Engl J Med.* 2016;**374**(6):523–532.

6. Knopman DS, Jack CR, Jr., Lundt ES, et al. Role of beta-amyloidosis and neurodegeneration in subsequent imaging changes in mild cognitive impairment. *JAMA Neurol.* 2015;**72**(12):1475–1483.

7. Brookmeyer R, Gray S, Kawas C. Projections of Alzheimer's disease in the United States and the public health impact of delaying disease onset. *Am J Public Health.* 1998;**88** (9):1337–1342.

8. Snowdon DA, Greiner LH, Mortimer JA, Riley KP, Greiner PA, Markesbery WR. Brain infarction and the clinical expression of Alzheimer disease: the Nun Study. *JAMA.* 1997;**277**(10):813–817.

9. Whitehead SN, Cheng G, Hachinski VC, Cechetto DF. Progressive increase in infarct size, neuroinflammation, and cognitive deficits in the presence of high levels of amyloid. *Stroke.* 2007;**38** (12):3245–3250.

10. Thiel A, Cechetto DF, Heiss WD, Hachinski V, Whitehead SN. Amyloid burden, neuroinflammation, and links to cognitive decline after ischemic stroke. *Stroke.* 2014;**45**(9):2825–2829.

11. Black SE. Vascular cognitive impairment: epidemiology, subtypes, diagnosis and management. *J R Coll Physicians Edinb.* 2011;**41**(1):49–56.

12. Hachinski V, Sposato LA. Dementia: from muddled diagnoses to treatable mechanisms. *Brain.* 2013;**136**(Pt 9): 2652–2624.

13. Hackam DG, Spence JD. Combining multiple approaches for the secondary prevention of vascular events after stroke: a quantitative modeling study. *Stroke.* 2007;**38**(6):1881–1885.

14. de Bruijn RF, Bos MJ, Portegies ML, et al. The potential for prevention of dementia across two decades: the prospective, population-based Rotterdam Study. *BMC Med.* 2015;**13**:132.

15. Chiuve SE, Rexrode KM, Spiegelman D, Logroscino G, Manson JE, Rimm EB. Primary prevention of stroke by healthy lifestyle. *Circulation.* 2008;**118**(9):947–954.

16. Larsson SC, Akesson A, Wolk A. Healthy diet and lifestyle and risk of stroke in a prospective cohort of women. *Neurology*. 2014;**83**(19):1699–1704.

17. Akesson A, Larsson SC, Discacciati A, Wolk A. Low-risk diet and lifestyle habits in the primary prevention of myocardial infarction in men: a population-based prospective cohort study. *J Am Coll Cardiol*. 2014;**64**(13):1299–1306.

18. Ngandu T, Lehtisalo J, Solomon A, et al. A 2 year multidomain intervention of diet, exercise, cognitive training, and vascular risk monitoring versus control to prevent cognitive decline in at-risk elderly people (FINGER): a randomised controlled trial. *Lancet*. 2015;**385**(9984):2255–2263.

19. Willett WC, Stampfer MJ. Rebuilding the food pyramid. *Sci Am*. 2003;**288**(1):64–71.

20. Keys A. Mediterranean diet and public health: personal reflections. *Am J Clin Nutr*. 1995;**61**(6 Suppl):1321S–1323S.

21. de Lorgeril M, Salen P, Martin JL, Monjaud I, Delaye J, Mamelle N. Mediterranean diet, traditional risk factors, and the rate of cardiovascular complications after myocardial infarction: final report of the Lyon Diet Heart Study. *Circulation*. 1999;**99**(6):779–785.

22. Estruch R, Ros E, Salas-Salvado J, Covas MI, Pharm D, Corella D, et al. Primary prevention of cardiovascular disease with a Mediterranean diet. *N Engl J Med*. 2013;**368**(14):1279–1290.

23. Valls-Pedret C, Sala-Vila A, Serra-Mir M, Corella D, de la Torre R, Martinez-Gonzalez MA, et al. Mediterranean diet and age-related cognitive decline: a randomized clinical trial. *JAMA Intern Med*. 2015;**175**(7):1094–1103.

24. Safouris A, Tsivgoulis G, Sergentanis TN, Psaltopoulou T. Mediterranean diet and risk of dementia. *Curr Alzheimer Res*. 2015;**12**(8):736–744.

25. Greger M. False and Misleading Claims by Egg Marketers. Available at http://nutritionfacts.org/video/eggs-and-cholesterol-patently-false-and-misleading-claims/. Accessed May 20, 2015.

26. Spence JD, Jenkins DJ, Davignon J. Dietary cholesterol and egg yolks: not for patients at risk of vascular disease. *Can J Cardiol*. 2010;**26**(9):e336–e339.

27. Reiner Z, Catapano AL, De BG, et al. ESC/EAS Guidelines for the management of dyslipidaemias: the task force for the management of dyslipidaemias of the European Society of Cardiology (ESC) and the European Atherosclerosis Society (EAS). *Eur Heart J*. 2011;**32**(14):1769–1818.

28. Spence JD. Fasting lipids: the carrot in the snowman. *Can J Cardiol*. 2003;**19**:890–892.

29. Spence JD, Jenkins DJ, Davignon J. Egg yolk consumption and carotid plaque. *Atherosclerosis*. 2012;**224**(2):469–73.

30. Spence JD, Jenkins DJA, Davignon J. Egg yolk consumption, smoking and carotid plaque: reply to letter to the editor. *Atherosclerosis*. 2013;**227**(1):189–191.

31. Wang Z, Klipfell E, Bennett BJ, et al. Gut flora metabolism of phosphatidylcholine promotes cardiovascular disease. *Nature*. 2011;**472**(7341):57–63.

32. Tang WHW, Wang Z, Levinson BS, et al. Intestinal microbiota metabolism of phosphatidylcholine and incident cardiac risks. *N Engl J Med*. 2013;**368**(17):1575–1584.

33. Spence JD. *How to prevent your stroke*. Nashville: Vanderbilt University Press; 2006.

34. Spence JD. Metabolic B12 deficiency: a missed opportunity to prevent dementia and stroke. *Nutr Res*. 2015;**36**(2):109–116.

35. Andres E, Loukili NH, Noel E, et al. Vitamin B12 (cobalamin) deficiency in elderly patients. *CMAJ*. 2004;**171**(3):251–259.

36. Spence JD. Nutrition and stroke prevention. *Stroke*. 2006;**37**(9):2430–2435.

37. Toole JF, Malinow MR, Chambless LE, et al. Lowering plasma total homocysteine to prevent recurrent stroke, myocardial infarction, and death in ischemic stroke patients: results of the Vitamin Intervention for Stroke Prevention (VISP)

randomized trial. *JAMA*. 2004;**291**(5):565–575.

38. Lonn E, Yusuf S, Arnold MJ, et al. Homocysteine lowering with folic acid and B vitamins in vascular disease. *N Engl J Med*. 2006;**354**(15):1567–1577.

39. Spence JD, Stampfer MJ. Understanding the complexity of homocysteine lowering with vitamins: the potential role of subgroup analyses. *JAMA*. 2011;**306**(23):2610–2611.

40. Spence JD, Bang H, Chambless LE, Stampfer MJ. Vitamin Intervention For Stroke Prevention trial: an efficacy analysis. *Stroke*. 2005;**36**(11):2404–2409.

41. House AA, Eliasziw M, Cattran DC, et al. Effect of b-vitamin therapy on progression of diabetic nephropathy: a randomized controlled trial. *JAMA*. 2010;**303**(16):1603–1609.

42. Spence JD, Eliasziw M, House AA. B-vitamin therapy for diabetic nephropathy: reply. *JAMA*. 2010;**304**(6):636–637.

43. Spence JD, Urquhart BL, Bang H. Effect of renal impairment on atherosclerosis: only partially mediated by homocysteine. *Nephrol Dial Transplant*. 2015;**31**(6):937–944.

44. Soros P, Whitehead S, Spence JD, Hachinski V. Antihypertensive treatment can prevent stroke and cognitive decline. *Nat Rev Neurol*. 2013;**9**(3):174–178.

45. Blanco P, Mueller L, Spence JD. Blood pressure gradients in cerebral arteries: a clue to pathogenesis of cerebral small vessel disease. *Stroke Vasc Neurol*. 2017;**0**: e000087.

46. Spence JD, Rayner BL. J curve and cuff artefact, and diagnostic inertia in resistant hypertension. *Hypertension*. 2016;**67**(1):32–33.

47. Howard G, Prineas R, Moy C, et al. Racial and geographic differences in awareness, treatment, and control of hypertension: the REasons for Geographic And Racial Differences in Stroke study. *Stroke*. 2006;**37**(5):1171–1178.

48. Spence JD. Lessons from Africa: the importance of measuring plasma renin and aldosterone in resistant hypertension. *Can J Cardiol*. 2012;**28**(3):254–257.

49. SPRINT Research Group. A randomized trial of intensive versus standard blood-pressure control. *N Engl J Med*. 2015;**373**(22):2103–2116.

50. McEvoy JW, Chen Y, Rawlings A, et al. Diastolic blood pressure, subclinical myocardial damage, and cardiac events: implications for blood pressure control. *J Am Coll Cardiol*. 2016;**68**(16): 1713–1722.

51. Hajjar I, Goldstein FC, Martin GS, Quyyumi AA. Roles of arterial stiffness and blood pressure in hypertension-associated cognitive decline in healthy adults. *Hypertension*. 2016;**67**(1):171–175.

52. Valdes Hernandez Mdel C, Maconick LC, Munoz Maniega S, et al. A comparison of location of acute symptomatic vs. 'silent' small vessel lesions. *Int J Stroke*. 2015;**10**(7):1044–1050.

53. Akintunde A, Nondi J, Gogo K, et al. Physiological phenotyping for personalized therapy of uncontrolled hypertension in Africa. *Am J Hypertens*. 2017;**30**(9):923–940.

54. Luchsinger JA, Lehtisalo J, Lindstrom J, et al. Cognition in the Finnish diabetes prevention study. *Diabetes Res Clin Pract*. 2015;**108**(3):e63–e66.

55. Grosser T, Fries S, Lawson JA, Kapoor SC, Grant GR, FitzGerald GA. Drug resistance and pseudoresistance: an unintended consequence of enteric coating aspirin. *Circulation*. 2013;**127**(3):377–385.

56. Spence JD, Hackam DG. Treating arteries instead of risk factors. a paradigm change in management of atherosclerosis. *Stroke*. 2010;**41**(6):1193–1199.

57. Spence JD, Coates V, Li H, et al. Effects of Intensive medical therapy on microemboli and cardiovascular risk in asymptomatic carotid stenosis. *Arch Neurol*. 2010;**67**(2):180–186.

58. Bogiatzi C, Spence JD. Ezetimibe and regression of carotid atherosclerosis: importance of measuring plaque burden. *Stroke*. 2012;**43**:1153–1155.

59. Spence JD. Management of asymptomatic carotid stenosis. *Neurol Clin.* 2015;**33**(2):443–457.

60. Spence JD. Management of patients with an asymptomatic carotid stenosis – medical management, endovascular treatment, or carotid endarterectomy? *Curr NeurolNeurosci Rep.* 2016; in press.

61. Gleason CE, Dowling NM, Wharton W, et al. Effects of hormone therapy on cognition and mood in recently postmenopausal women: findings from the randomized, controlled KEEPS-Cognitive and Affective Study. *PLoS Med.* 2015;**12**(6): e1001833; discussion e.

62. Marjoribanks J, Farquhar C, Roberts H, Lethaby A. Long term hormone therapy for perimenopausal and postmenopausal women. *Cochrane Database Syst Rev.* 2012;7:CD004143.

63. Lv W, Du N, Liu Y, et al. Low testosterone level and risk of Alzheimer's disease in the elderly men: a systematic review and meta-analysis. *Mol Neurobiol.* 2016 ;**53**(4):2679–2684.

64. Spence JD, Pilote L. Importance of sex and gender in atherosclerosis and cardiovascular disease. *Atherosclerosis.* 2015;**241**(1):208–210.

65. Sharma R, Oni OA, Gupta K, et al. Normalization of testosterone level is associated with reduced incidence of myocardial infarction and mortality in men. *Eur Heart J.* 2015;**36**(40):2706–2715.

Conclusion

Vladimir Hachinski

Although the emphasis of this book has been on cognitive impairment and its prevention, there is a sunny side to brain health, namely resilience, which can be defined as physical robustness and mental fortitude. Many still unknown factors remain to be discovered. However, social contacts and support, physical and mental activity, and a healthy attitude towards life all contribute to resilience. Probably, in the future we will understand better the interaction of mechanisms that impair cognition versus those that preserve it and enhance it.

Typically, diseases have been described and studied in isolation, with the emphasis on distinctive characteristics; with aging these distinctions become increasingly blurred, especially in relation to the brain. A trend is arising towards addressing mechanisms common to all major neurological diseases, such as inflammation, oxidative stress, neurotransmission failure excitotoxicity, and apoptosis. It is likely that in the future there will be multiple drugs attacking interactive mechanisms that may be helpful, not only in stroke, but in Alzheimer pathology and other neurodegenerative disorders.

The future, probably will also bring personalized medicine. Individual patients will not only have their health profile documented, but also their genetic predisposition to diseases and reaction to medications so that their care can be individualized. Messages to patients so that they follow advice may have to be tailored, not only to what stage of decision making they find themselves in, but also to their particular personality type.

John Donne wrote that "no man is an island," nor are women. This is particularly true when it comes to the management of risk factors and the encouragement of healthy lifestyles. Clearly, it is much easier for an individual to have healthy lifestyles if the environment in which he/she has grown up is healthy and also whether there is a supportive community and urban planning that allows for this. This needs to be supplemented by national and international policies that foster healthy lifestyle and have an effective health care system to deal with patients when they become ill.

The road ahead will remain arduous because we will need to shed some of the conceptual baggage that we now carry and also expand up our interventions from the clinic and hospitals to a presymptomatic stage where physicians act as advisors and leaders. Greater responsibility needs to be taken by individuals for their health with technological support and individualization in allowing for a healthy lifestyle. Similarly, when something goes wrong, it is likely that with smart technology and algorithms, it may be possible to detect problems earlier and deal with them more effectively.

Cognitive impairment is not a threshold but a continuum. It is caused by multiple interactive pathologies among which vascular disease is the most prevalent and the only treatable and preventable one. It is encouraging that in some of the countries where the incidence of stroke has declined dementia incidence tends to follow, presumably in part due to healthier lifestyles and control of risk factors and preventing stroke itself, that triples the risk of developing dementia.

The future will be different, and probably better.

Vladimir Hachinski

Index